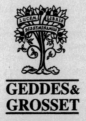

GEDDES & GROSSET

This edition published by Geddes & Grosset, an imprint of
Children's Leisure Products Limited

© 1998 Children's Leisure Products Limited,
David Dale House, New Lanark ML11 9DJ, Scotland

Cover photograph by Nicholas Rigg courtesy of the
Telegraph Colour Library

First published 1998
Reprinted 1999

ISBN 1 85534 337 1

Printed and bound in the UK

Contents

Identifying the Problem: Diagnosis

It can be exceedingly difficult, even for doctors, to make a diagnosis at times of emergency without the support of hospital testing facilities. Often it will be impossible for the first-aider to obtain a reliable history from the patient if he or she is unconscious or severely shocked. If the first-aider is confident that he or she can identify life-threatening conditions in the first instance then detailed history-taking is of secondary importance. Where a patient is unable to give details of events leading up to an accident or emergency, then this information should be sought from any relations or bystanders who might be able to provide useful information. Wherever possible, the first-aider should try to ascertain the patient's name and age and whether or not he or she has any significant medical problems or is currently taking any medication for a specific condition.

At the Scene of the Emergency

Before dealing with any patient in need of first aid, it is important to check that you will not actually exacerbate the situation or put yourself at risk. It is vital that you send for specialist help as soon as possible – for this you may be able to use bystanders after instructing them clearly which emergency services you require. You may need to be aware of the safety implications of dealing with a patient in conditions such as heavy traffic or fire, circumstances that will always require increased levels of calm and concentration. You must never be afraid to admit your limitations as a first-aider and should always be prepared to make way for professionals.

Bites and Stings

When an insect, such as a bee, a wasp or a hornet, stings it injects a tiny amount of venom beneath the skin, causing localised swelling and redness. Although painful, insect stings are rarely serious and the symptoms will begin to subside after 3–4 hours. However, stings can be dangerous, even fatal, if the individual is allergic to the venom or if he has suffered multiple stings. In this case it is essential that the victim receives medical attention immediately.

Insect stings

1 Only honey bees will actually leave their sting embedded in the skin. If the sting is visible, then carefully remove it with the edge of a knife or fingernail. Do not squeeze the sting as this will release more venom.

2 Wash the sting site with soap and water and apply ice wrapped in cloth or a cold compress to the area for up to 30 minutes to reduce the swelling.

bee sting removal

Allergic Reaction to an Insect Sting
1 Swelling around the face or on other parts of the body.
2 Difficulty with breathing and swallowing.
3 Weakness and dizziness.
4 Nausea and stomach cramps.
5 Unconsciousness.

To treat an allergic reaction
1 Lie the casualty still and ensure that the stung limb is lower than the level of the heart.
2 Seek emergency medical help immediately.

Animal Bites
Bites which have been caused by an animal or a human should always be referred for medical examination because there is a risk that bacteria on teeth and in saliva will lead to infection.

Bleeding can be quite severe depending upon the type and number of bites, and the first-aider's initial aim should be to control the bleeding.

Treatment for a superficial wound

1 If bleeding is not severe then wash the wound thoroughly with soap and water to try to remove some of the possible contamination.
2 Control bleeding by applying a sterile dressing or a clean pad and pressing it firmly against the wound.
3 When bleeding has ceased, cover the wound with a fresh dressing held in place with adhesive tape or bandaging.
4 Seek medical examination of the wound. **Do not** apply medicated ointment to the wound.

Treatment for a severe wound

1 Arrange for the prompt removal of the casualty to hospital.
2 Control serious bleeding by applying direct pressure to the wound(s).
3 Cover the wound with a sterile dressing or a pad of clean cloth.
4 Observe the casualty for signs of shock.

Snakebites

Snakebites are rarely fatal but the venom which is released in the bite can cause considerable pain to the victim and may result in illness. It is, therefore, essential that a snakebite receives medical examination as soon as possible.

The adder is the only poisonous snake that is indigenous to Britain – a snake kept in a zoo or as part of a private collection is likely to be of foreign origin and it must always be assumed that such a snake is poisonous.

Treatment for a snakebite

1 Identify the snake if possible and pass this information on to medical staff at the nearest casualty department immediately – this will enable them to identify and prepare the appropriate anti-venom.
2 Before the casualty is transported to hospital, particularly if the journey will take some time, it is important to reduce the amount of venom in the bite wound and inhibit the spread of the venom in the body. Wash the wound with soap and water if possible and cover it with a dressing or a clean cloth. Place a broad bandage just above the site of the wound and fix it firmly but not too tightly in place to make a ligature.
3 Immobilise the affected limb with a splint if possible.
4 Reassure the casualty and observe for signs of shock. Administer mild analgesics such as paracetamol and aspirin if necessary.
6 Arrange for the casualty's immediate removal to hospital.

Bleeding

Blood is the medium in which oxygen is carried to all the living tissues of the body. Therefore, the loss of any great quantity of blood represents a threat to life itself and should always be treated as a medical emergency. The body has a very sophisticated clotting mechanism that can seal up small lesions quickly and efficiently. Furthermore, a healthy adult may suffer no ill effects even after a loss of 850 ml or $1\frac{1}{2}$ pints.

The difficulty in an emergency situation is that it is often impossible to assess accurately the volume of blood that has been lost. It is therefore advisable for the first-aider to take prompt action to stop bleeding wherever possible.

The type of bleeding suffered by a patient will be dependent on the type of wound sustained. An open wound is one in which there is a visible break in the skin, whereas a closed wound causes the escape of blood from the circulation into the body tissues. The first kind of bleeding is known as **external** bleeding, and the second is known as **internal** bleeding.

Emergency Action for Bleeding

Wherever possible, try to be aware of your own safety. If you have any open wounds, try to ensure that there is a barrier between yourself and the casualty's wound before dealing with bleeding.

1 Locate and examine the wound for foreign bodies such as glass. Remove any clothing obstructing your access to the wound. If the wound appears to be free of glass, etc, apply pressure directly onto the wound. If the wound is long, or there is a foreign body protruding from it, press down firmly on either side of the wound whilst trying to keep the edges as close together as possible. Apply pressure with a clean pad of material or sterile dressing, but this is not essential and it is important not to waste time searching for one.

2 Elevate the affected part above the level of the patient's heart – you may find it easier to lie the patient down. **Do not** handle a limb you suspect

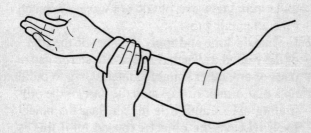

elevate the affected part above the patient's heart

may be fractured other than attempting to stop
bleeding.
3 Continue to apply pressure for at least 10 minutes. If your original pad or dressing has become
saturated, do not remove it. If possible wrap more
bandages round it firmly, but not so tightly as to
obstruct circulation. Scarves, clean sheets and
handkerchiefs, etc, make suitable substitutes for
bandages.

If the wound contains a foreign body:
1 Make no attempt to pull out the foreign body as

this could exacerbate bleeding and shock – it may be acting as a partial 'plug'. However, if it appears loose, it may be possible to flush it out under running water, but do not waste too much time attempting this.

2 Elevate the limb and apply pressure on the edges of the wound. If you have access to sterile gauze pads or any other suitable material, try to build up a platform or ring around the base of the protruding object until it is higher than the object itself. (Leave the object exposed until this is achieved.)

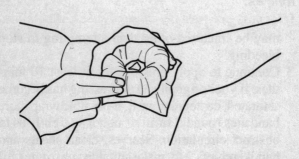

if the wound contains a foreign body elevate the limb and apply pressure on the edges of the wound

3 Bandage firmly on either side of the wound, but avoiding the wound and the embedded object.
4 Cover the wound loosely with sterile dressings or clean material, elevate the limb and **seek medical help immediately**.

Remember – your priorities are:
1 To control bleeding and prevent shock (*see* p.100).
2 To prevent or minimise infection.
3 To secure medical help for your patient as quickly as possible.

If despite your best efforts the patient begins to display symptoms of shock, then treat as follows:
1 Identify and treat the cause of shock, if possible.
2 Lay the patient flat on the floor as comfortably as possible.
3 Elevate his or her legs above head height (unless you suspect a fracture).
4 Loosen any restrictive articles of clothing.
5 Keep the patient warm by covering with blankets, rugs or coats, but do not apply a direct heat source such as a hot-water bottle.
6 Keep a check on the patient's vital signs – pulse and respiration – and level of consciousness. Be ready to resuscitate if necessary (*see* ABC of Resuscitation on p.71).

Internal Bleeding

Internal bleeding may result from injury such as bone fracture or severe bruising, but it can also occur spontaneously as the result of a stomach ulcer or vaginal bleeding or several other medical emergencies. In the absence of any visible blood, the diagnosis is often a hard one to make, but signs and symptoms of shock (*see* p.100) will emerge if internal bleeding is significant. Sometimes there will be blood present at body orifices, and there may be bruising. Always treat for shock and summon medical help immediately.

Nosebleeds

Nosebleeds are rarely serious and most commonly occur either after a blow to the nose, as part of an infection such as the common cold, or as a consequence of picking or blowing the nose. Occasionally, frequent nosebleeds may be a result of high blood pressure or a sign of a weak blood vessel inside the nose that ruptures spontaneously from time to time. Normally, nosebleeds are simply inconvenient and unpleasant, but occasionally they can be dangerous if bleeding is prolonged, as the casualty can suffer considerable blood loss perhaps resulting in shock. If the blood coming from the nose appears thin and watery, summon medical help immediately, as this may indicate leakage of fluid from around the brain as a result of head or facial injury.

To Treat a Nosebleed

1 Seat the patient comfortably with the head forward. Do not tip the head back in an attempt to stop bleeding, as the patient will be forced to swallow the blood as it trickles down the back of his or her throat, which may cause vomiting.

2 Pinch the patient's nose just beneath the bridge and ask him or her to breathe through the mouth.

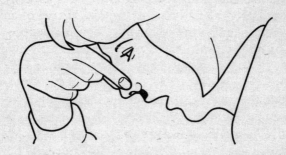

pinch the patient's nose just beneath the bridge and ask her to breathe through the mouth

3 Ask the casualty not to speak, sniff or swallow if possible as this may hinder clots from forming.

4 Apply pressure for a full 10 minutes in the first instance. If bleeding persists, apply a further 10 minutes' pressure. If bleeding has not ceased completely within 30 minutes, consult a doctor immediately or take the patient to the nearest accident and emergency unit. The patient should remain in the treatment position while travelling.

5 If bleeding stops, clean gently around the nose with cotton wool or a swab soaked in warm water. Ask the patient not to blow his or her nose for at least four hours and to rest quietly to avoid dislodging the clot.

Breathing Difficulties

Asthma

Asthma is an increasingly common respiratory disorder that can be triggered by allergy, exertion, cigarette smoke, respiratory infection or by emotional factors. The patient will experience increasing tightness in the chest and difficulty in breathing as the air passages constrict. Breathing is characterised by wheezing, which may be audible as a whistling sound, particularly when the patient breathes out. Most asthma sufferers cope well with the problem, and will usually be aware of the onset of an attack and take appropriate medication, usually in the form of inhalers. However, if it is the patient's first attack and he or she does not have medication, or if medication has been taken but without any response, it is essential that medical help is summoned immediately as asthma can be fatal.

Symptoms of an asthmatic attack

1 Difficulty in breathing, anxiety and difficulty in speaking.
2 Blueish appearance to the face, especially around the lips.

To treat an attack of asthma

1 Sit the patient at a table and encourage him or her to lean forward with the arms resting on the top of a table.
2 Ensure the room has an adequate supply of fresh air. Open a window, but not if the weather is cold.
3 Reassure the patient and encourage him or her to take his or her medication.
4 If there has been no response to the inhaler within 10 or 15 minutes, or if the patient becomes drowsy or begins to go blue around the lips, telephone for an ambulance immediately.

Croup

Croup is a breathing disorder of very young children caused by inflammation of the trachea (windpipe) and larynx. It is characterised by a barking cough, perhaps accompanied by a wheezing or whistling sound (known as **stridor**), and in severe cases the child may appear blue. It frequently occurs at night and can be very alarming, but an at-

tack almost always resolves itself without further
problems. Recovery can be quickened by:

1 Taking the child into a steam-filled room, such
  as a bathroom with the hot tap running in the
  bath.
2 Keeping the atmosphere in the child's bedroom
  humid.

It is advisable to call your doctor as the condition can recur after the initial attack has subsided.

If the child is sitting bolt upright or has a high
temperature, this may indicate a more serious condition, known as **epiglottitis,** which requires immediate medical attention.

Hyperventilation

Hyperventilation occurs when an individual experiences an emotional fright, upset or stress. It is
characterised by a shallow, rapid breathing pattern,
whereby too much carbon dioxide is removed from
the body. This causes feelings of dizziness and tingling, and may cause the individual to panic. Adequate carbon dioxide levels can be restored and
the symptoms controlled by encouraging the individual to breath into a paper bag held over his or
her nose and mouth for up to four minutes.

Burns and Scalds

Burns are sustained in a number of ways – most commonly from dry heat, friction or corrosive chemicals – whilst scalds are caused by liquids and vapours. Although heat accounts for most burns and scalds, it is important to remember that contact with extreme cold can also burn, as can radiation.

At the scene of the burns incident:

1 Make sure you do not put yourself in danger from the presence of fire, electrical hazards, etc.
2 Where possible, stop the burning of affected tissues by rapid cooling. The most effective way of doing this is to place the affected limb or part under cold running water **for at least 10 minutes**. This will help to minimise tissue damage, swelling, shock and pain.

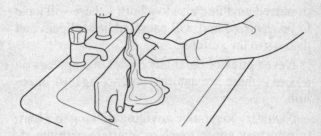

*the most effective way of rapid cooling is to place
the affected part under cold running water
for **at least 10 minutes***

3 If removing the patient to hospital, turn off the
water and cover the wound. A **non-stick** sterile
dressing is preferable, but if not available, a clean
handkerchief, pillowcase or sheet will do. Burns
are highly vulnerable to infection, so it is important not to leave a wound exposed to the atmosphere for any length of time.

4 Keep the patient as calm as possible and observe
for signs of shock (*see* p.100). Always obtain
medical help quickly for all but the most minor
of burns.

25

Never use an adhesive dressing on a burn.

Never apply creams, ointments, sprays, butter, or indeed anything else to a burn – these will have to be removed and will cause additional pain and distress to the sufferer.

Never prick or burst any blister that appears on a burn – these are nature's defence against infection.

Never try to remove anything sticking to a burn – in fact try not to touch or interfere with the affected area at all.

Burns to the Mouth and Throat

Burns on the face and mouth are extremely serious as they can cause rapid swelling of the airways. Summon medical help immediately and be prepared to resuscitate. Inform the ambulance service that you suspect burns of the airway.

Electrical burns

Burns may be caused by an electrical current passing into the body. Although most damage is done at the points of entry and exit, occasionally tracks of damage are caused internally. Severe electric shock may cause cardiac arrest – if the victim is unconscious, disregard any burns initially and give priority to the ABC of Resuscitation (*see* p.71).

If the source of electricity is low voltage, such as from the domestic supply, it is essential to isolate the casualty from the current, either by disconnecting the power or using wood or plastic to separate the victim from the appliance. Alternatively, wrench the cable from the plug or grab the victims clothing and pull him or herher free. **Do not come into contact with the victim's skin**.

Thereafter
1 Treat the site of injury as for any other burn.
2 Observe and treat the victim for shock and summon an ambulance.

Chemical burns
Chemicals that cause severe burns are normally found in industry, but some paint strippers and other domestic chemicals can also inflict similar burns. Try to find out what the substance was in order to inform the doctor, and summon medical help immediately. In the meantime:
1 Flood the burnt area with copious amounts of running water. Protect yourself with rubber gloves.
2 Remove any clothing that is likely to be contaminated with the chemical.
3 Get the casualty to hospital as quickly as possible.

Chemical Burns to the Eyes

If the eyes are affected, it is essential to pour as much water into them as possible. This will obviously need to be done as gently as possible, and as the eyes will probably be tightly shut in pain, it may be necessary to prise them open firmly. Chemical burns to the eyes can cause lasting damage, and even blindness, so it is essential to seek hospital treatment without delay.

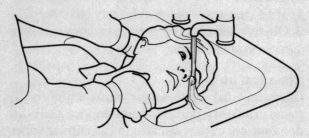

with chemical burns to the eyes it is essential to pour gently as much water into the eyes as possible

Choking

Normally when we swallow, a flap of cartilage, known as the epiglottis, moves downwards to stop food being taken into the trachea, or windpipe. Where this fails to happen, food becomes stuck in the airway and choking is said to have occurred. Sometimes the victim may appear to vomit or cough up the foreign body, but occasionally this fails to happen and the patient may be unable to breathe, either partially or completely. Where a choking victim is unable to breathe, action must be taken immediately, as brain damage will occur within three or four minutes of its being starved of oxygen. Choking is a common cause of accidental death amongst children.

How to Recognise a Choking Attack

1 The victim will probably clutch at his or her throat and be unable to speak.

2 The victim will probably become acutely distressed and panicky.

3 Inability to breathe will probably result in fairly rapid loss of consciousness.

Emergency Action for a Choking Attack in an Adult

1 Lean the victim forwards and give him or her five hard slaps on the back between the shoulder blades.

2 If this is unsuccessful, then abdominal thrusts can be performed from behind a patient who is either standing or sitting. For this, pass your hands around the patient and interlock your hands together just above the navel in the region of the diaphragm and pull sharply inwards and upwards (also known as the Heimlech's manoevre).

3 If the casualty is unconscious, kneel astride him or her on the floor and perform similar abdominal thrusts with the heel of the hand (one hand positioned on top of the other) just below the rib-cage

4 If you have tried abdominal thrusts six times without response, telephone 999 for an ambulance and begin resuscitation immediately (*see* p. 71).

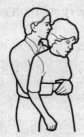 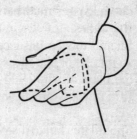

pass your hands around the patient, interlock your hands together just above the navel in the region of the diaphragm and pull sharply inwards and upwards

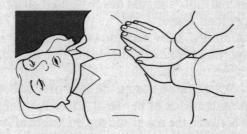

if the casualty is unconscious, kneel astride her on the floor and perform similar abdominal thrusts with the heel of the hand just below the rib cage

Emergency Action for a Choking Child

1 Lay the child across your lap with his or her head down. Slap firmly between the shoulder blades five times.
2 Should this be unsuccessful, turn the child over so that he or she faces you on your lap. Support the back of the child and give him or her five firm upward thrusts with one hand above the navel.
3 Should this fail to dislodge the foreign body, then try steps 1 and 2 again. If the child becomes unconscious, then call an ambulance immediately and begin resuscitation (*see* p. 71 and 79).

Emergency Action for a Choking Baby

Abdominal thrusts should **never** be used on a child younger than 1 year.
1 Straddle the baby face down along your arm suuporting her head and give her five firm slaps between the shoulders.
2 If choking continues, turn the baby over, still supporting the back of her head. Place two fingertips between the navel and the breastbone. Press forward and downward in quick movements and repeat the movement up to four times if necessary.
3 If the infant loses consciousness, summon medi-

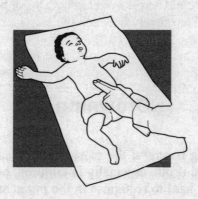

• *place two fingertips between the navel and the breastbone*
• *press forward and downward in quick movements*
• *repeat movement up to four times if necessary*

cal help immediately and begin resuscitation (*see* page 71).

Remember:

Never poke your fingers down a choking victim's throat in an attempt to find the obstructing object – you will only push it in further and make it more difficult to dislodge. If the object appears in or at the victim's mouth, then you may remove it gently.

Drowning

Drowning is one of the most common causes of accidental death, especially in children, but is often quite hard to recognise in the initial stages. It may be very hard for a person drowning to summon the energy to shout, so the sight of a swimmer waving should always be treated with suspicion. The victim will attempt to hold his or her breath for as long as possible but will eventually be forced to take a breath, permitting water to enter the airway. The muscles in the throat will respond by going into spasm, which will then restrict breathing. The patient will quickly lapse into unconsciousness as the oxygen supply to the brain is cut off.

The brain will sustain permanent damage after it has been deprived of oxygen for just three or four minutes, unless the water is very cold. Under these circumstances, the brain may require less oxygen and may survive unharmed for up to 30 minutes or more, particularly in the case of children. Therefore, it is always worth resuscitating a victim who has been pulled from cold water, even if you suspect he or she has been submerged for longer than four minutes.

Rescue and Treatment of a Drowning Victim

1 **Do not risk your own safety**. Try to reach the victim from land by extending a pole or a rope. **Do not** attempt to swim or wade through a strong current or deep, cold water as you may find yourself quickly overcome.

2 If you are carrying the victim to safety, try to ensure that you have a floating object, such as a board or a lifebelt, that he or she can grab hold of; in panic the victim may grab you and thus make it more difficult for you to keep afloat. Keep his or her head tilted below the level of the body to allow as much water to drain naturally as possible. Similarly, when laying the victim down, try to do so on a slope with the head downmost.

3 Check the airway for signs of obstruction with weeds or other debris, and clear by using finger sweeps, except in very small children. **Do not** use abdominal thrusts as this may cause stomach contents to be inhaled.

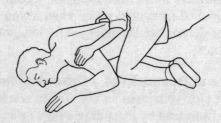

*when laying the victim down, try to do so on a slope
with his head downmost*

4 If the victim still has a carotid pulse but is fail-
ing to breathe, then begin mouth-to-mouth ventilation straight away (*see* p.74).

5 If there is no carotid pulse or breathing, then send
someone for an ambulance and give full cardiopulmonary resuscitation (*see* p.76).

6 Even though your patient appears to have made
a full recovery, always send him to hospital for
observation as serious breathing difficulties may
recur some hours after the accident. Whilst awaiting the arrival of the emergency services, keep
the patient as warm as possible, as he may be
suffering from hypothermia.

Fainting and Fits

Epilepsy

Epilepsy is a common condition in which the sufferer experiences a fit or seizure in response to sudden disruption of normal electrical activity in the brain. In an attack, the casualty may suddenly fall to the ground unconscious. For a few seconds, the muscles may stiffen and breathing will stop. This is known as the **tonic** phase, and it is succeeded by the **clonic** phase, in which the whole body jerks violently and breathing recommences noisily through clenched teeth. Normally, the jerking will cease and the muscles relax within about a minute. Breathing will become normal again, but the patient may remain unconscious for a few more minutes.

Although epileptic fits can be frightening to witness, they rarely cause the sufferers any lasting harm, unless they have injured themselves during the fall or the clonic phase.

How to Help During an Epileptic Fit

1 Move furniture and other objects to clear a space around the patient and, if possible, position him or her on the back before the jerking begins.

2 Loosen tight clothing, but do not attempt to restrain the patient or put anything in the mouth during the attack.

3 When the convulsion has subsided, place the patient in the recovery position (*see* p.83) and remain with him or her until a complete recovery has been made.

4 Examine the patient for signs of injury, such as cuts or fractures. When the patient is fit to move, ensure that he or she gets home safely and informs a doctor, especially if this is the first attack.

5 If the patient does not regain consciousness within 15 minutes or has repeated convulsions, then call an ambulance.

Fainting

Fainting is a temporary loss of consciousness occasioned by a reduced blood supply to the brain. This may be caused by an emotional shock, fear, pain or inadequate food intake over a period of time. More usually, however, people faint after long spells of inactivity, particularly in warm, airless conditions, during which blood will tend to pool in the lower part of the body, thereby reducing the amount available to the brain.

Treatment of fainting:

1 Lie the casualty down on the floor and raise the legs above the level of the head.
2 Open the windows and wait for the casualty to regain consciousness – usually within a few minutes.
3 If the patient recovers, but continues to feel faint, ask him or her to sit with the head down between the knees.
4 If the casualty does not regain consciousness quickly, place him or her in the recovery position (*see* p.83), check pulse and respiration, and call for an ambulance. Be prepared to resuscitate if necessary.

Febrile Convulsion

Febrile convulsions are caused by overheating and are most common in children under two. There is usually a history of fever and illness, such as throat infection, which is often exacerbated by the child being wrapped too warmly in bed. Typically, the child's skin will be flushed and hot, and the convulsion is characterised by arching of the back and violent muscle-twitching. The fists may be clenched and the eyes rolled upwards, and the breath is often held.

Treatment of a febrile convulsion is aimed at reducing the child's body temperature.

1 Remove the child's blankets and clothing.
2 Sponge the child with a sponge or flannel soaked in tepid water, starting from the head and working downwards.
3 Keep the airway open by placing the child in the recovery position (*see* p.83).
4 Pad around the child with soft pillows to prevent him or her from hurting himself or herself during a convulsion.
5 Call the doctor.

Foreign Bodies

Foreign Body in the Nose
A foreign body that is lodged in the nose should always receive medical attention. Attempts to remove the object, particularly if it is sharp, may cause damage to the tissue.

Signs and symptoms
1 The casualty will appear to have some difficulty in breathing through the nose.
2 Bleeding or discharge from one or both nostrils will be apparent.
3 The nose may be swollen.

Treatment
1 Advise the patient to breathe through the mouth.
2 Reassure the patient and arrange for him to receive medical attention as soon as possible.

Foreign Body in the Ear

As with foreign bodies in the nose, this type of injury is often sustained by young children. In most cases no attempt should be made to remove the foreign body as this may cause serious injury to the delicate eardrum; it is essential that the casualty receives medical attention as soon as possible.

Signs and symptoms

1 The patient may complain of impaired hearing in the affected ear.
2 The patient will complain of pain or discomfort in the ear.

Foreign Body in the Eye

Foreign bodies in the eye are fairly common. Eyelashes or small particles of dust, sand or grit often become lodged underneath the eyelid or stuck to the surface of the eyeball. While these can cause the casualty discomfort and the eye tissue to become inflamed, they are usually quite easily removed. However, if a foreign body is embedded in the eyeball or is on the iris, then no attempt should be made to remove it; in such cases the casualty should always receive medical treatment.

Signs and symptoms

1 The casualty will complain of discomfort and will probably attempt to rub the affected eye.
2 The affected eye will appear red and inflamed and will water.
3 The patient may complain that vision is impaired.

Treatment

1 Discourage the patient from rubbing the eye and reassure him or her.
2 If possible, sit the casualty in a chair and ask him or her to lean the head back.
3 Examine the casualty's eye, supporting the chin with one hand and using the other hand (index finger and thumb) to open the eye wide by stretching the upper and lower lid. If you ask the casualty to move the eyeball up and down, and from left to right, you will be able to examine the eyeball more effectively.
4 If you can locate the foreign body, try to remove it by washing it out with distilled water or fresh tap water if this is not available. Lean the head over on the affected side so that the water runs away down the cheek. If water is not readily accessible, then try to use a moistened swab, such as the corner of a damp, clean handkerchief.

5 If the foreign body is embedded on the iris (the coloured area of the eye) or cannot be removed using steps 1 to 4, then the casualty should receive medical attention. Try to cover the eye with a sterile dressing (ideally an eye pad) and secure it in place, ensuring that there is not too much pressure applied to the eyeball

6 Arrange for the casualty to be removed to hospital.

Ingested Foreign Bodies

A foreign body that has been swallowed may, if sharp, cause choking or result in damage being caused to the gastro-intestinal tract. Never attempt to make the casualty vomit as a method of removing the object – this will inevitably result in much greater damage and distress.

If the casualty has swallowed a foreign object, then it is important to ascertain precisely what the object is and to remove the casualty to hospital as soon as possible. Do not allow the patient to take anything by mouth, provide reassurance and observe for signs of discomfort.

Fractures

A fracture is a crack or break in a bone. It takes a considerable degree of force to break bones as they are not simply brittle sticks but living tissues supporting the body. However, the bones of the elderly or those affected by disease may become more brittle and vulnerable, whilst those of children may be more likely to split under force as they are more supple. Bones are supplied with a rich network of nerves and blood vessels, which accounts for the amount of pain and swelling experienced when a fracture is sustained.

Types of Fracture
1 **Simple fracture**: a clean break in a bone.
2 **Compound fracture**: a break in which the broken bone pierces the skin or is accompanied by a wound. In a compound fracture, the bone is exposed to contamination by infection from the air.

3 **Comminuted fracture**: the bone is shattered into several fragments at the site of the break.
4 **Greenstick fracture**: most commonly experienced by children. This type of fracture will show up on an X-ray as an incomplete break or split in a bone.
5 **Pathological fracture**: the bone may break spontaneously where affected by disease or some other weakening factor such as a cyst.

Signs and Symptoms of Fracture

1 The patient may report having heard or felt a snap, although this can be caused by injuries other than fracture.
2 The patient will often experience severe pain that is worsened by attempts to move the limb.
3 The patient will be unable to move the limb normally as a result of the pain and the instability of the broken bone.
4 Bleeding from the damaged bone and surrounding tissues will quickly result in swelling. Some time later, bruising will probably occur, again as a result of haemorrhage within the tissues.
5 The limb may be misshapen or deformed as a result of the break, or thrown into an unnatural position.

How to help a fracture victim

1 With the exception of suspected fractures to small bones in the upper limbs, it is best not to move the casualty, especially if you suspect the spine may be fractured.

2 Steady the broken limb by holding it gently but firmly above and below the fracture site, but do not attempt to straighten it.

3 Dial 999 for an ambulance at the earliest possible opportunity.

4 It may be possible to immobilise the injured part without moving it unduly. For example, it may be possible to support a broken leg between two cushions or pads of folded clothing, but do not attempt this if it involves moving the limb or altering its position. It is always a good idea to immobilise a broken arm against the body, using a sling (*see* page 65).

5 If it looks as if help may be some time in arriving, a broken leg may be gently secured to the sound leg with bandages. However, do not persist with this if it seems to be causing additional pain or distress.

6 Reassure the patient and observe for shock (*see* p.100)

7 Keep the patient warm, but do not give him or her anything to eat or drink, as he or she may

require a general anaesthetic on admission to hospital.

Open Fractures

Open fractures (i.e. those in which the broken bone is exposed to the air through a wound in the skin) should be treated in much the same way as closed fractures. The main problem is that as the wound is open, it is more prone to infection and there may be considerable blood loss. As with any fracture, it is essential to arrange for early removal of the casualty to hospital. Whilst waiting for the ambulance to arrive, proceed as follows:

1 Support the wound in the same way as you would with a closed fracture.
2 Gently cover the wound with a sterile dressing or clean pad of material.
3 Place more padding such as cotton wool around the pad and build it high enough to prevent pressure on any protruding bone (*see* p.16).
4 Bandage the padding gently but firmly in place. Take care not to bandage it so tightly that it impedes circulation or causes the patient further pain.
5 If possible, elevate and immobilise the limb.
6 Reassure the patient and observe for shock (*see* p.100).

Facial fractures

Broken noses, cheekbones and jaws are among the most common injuries to the face. The main problems with injuries of this type is that the airway may become blocked by swelling or bleeding, or perhaps by teeth that have been dislodged. Bear in mind that the blow that caused the most obvious injury may also have caused damage to the skull, the neck or even the brain.

Injuries/Fractures of the Nose and Cheekbones

These injuries frequently occur as a result of fighting and can cause considerable discomfort as swelling progresses. The aim of the first-aider is to reduce the swelling and to have the patient examined in hospital as soon as possible. Treat swelling as follows:

1 Apply a cold compress. (A flannel or large handkerchief soaked in cold water then frequently refreshed will suit this purpose.)
2 Take or send the patient to hospital.

Fracture of the Lower Jaw

This injury is usually caused by direct force to the jaw, either by a blow or a heavy fall. The pain can be excruciating and is often exacerbated by movement of the jaw, which is often hard to avoid. Fast removal of the patient to hospital is vital, but in the meantime you can make him or her more comfortable.

1 Encourage her to sit upright with her head tilted forward. This will encourage blood and saliva to drain from the mouth rather than necessitating swallowing.

2 Give the patient a soft pad and allow her to hold it in place against the painful jaw to support it. Encourage her to keep the jaw supported or tie a narrow bandage around the head until she reaches the hospital.

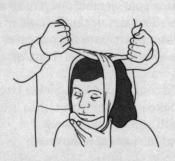

• give the patient a soft pad and allow her to hold it in place to support the jaw
• tie a narrow bandage around the head until she reaches the hospital

If the Facial Injury Victim is Unconscious
1 Check frequently that the airway is clear.
2 Place the patient in the recovery position (*see* p.83).
3 Call an ambulance immediately.
4 If a fractured jaw is suspected, slip a pad of soft material under the head in order to prevent its weight resting on and further damaging the jaw.

Remember that an injury above chest level should be treated as a suspected spinal injury (*see* page 60).

Fractures of the Upper Limb
The term 'upper limb' includes not only the arm but also the shoulder and the collarbone. If the patient can walk without too much distress, then it may be unnecessary to call an ambulance, although hospital treatment is essential.

Fracture of the Collarbone
The collarbone is situated at the base of the neck and supplies the arm's support between the breastbone and the shoulder blade. Fractures are usually a result of indirect force, such as an outstretched hand during a fall transmitting the force up to the collarbone. The patient will undoubtedly experience pain at the injury site, and will frequently at-

tempt to relieve this by tilting the head to one side.
If a fractured collar-bone is suspected:

1 Immobilise the arm on the injured side by sitting the patient down and placing the arm on the affected side across the chest, with the fingertips resting lightly on the opposite shoulder.

2 Place some padding between the injured limb and the casualty's chest. Support the arm in this position in an elevation sling across the shoulder (*see* p.67).

3 Give the arm further support if possible by adding an additional broadfold bandage around the chest.

4 Take the patient to hospital.

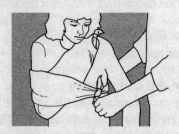

- *place the arm on the affected side across the chest*
  with fingertips resting on the opposite shoulder
  - *support with an elevation sling*
- *give the arm further support by adding an additional*
  broadfold bandage around the chest

Dislocation of the Shoulder

Dislocation of the shoulder is most commonly caused by a fall. In dislocation, the ball-type shoulder joint is wrenched out of its socket, causing extreme pain, especially upon movement. The first-aider's main aim is to reduce the pain by immobilising the joint until the casualty can be taken to hospital – **do not** attempt to relocate the joint. Seat the patient then:

1 Gently position the affected arm across the chest and apply an arm sling (*see* p.65).
2 Slip some padding behind the sling to give further support on the affected side. Check that the sling is not too tight by feeling for the pulse or numbness in the fingers
3 Arrange for the patient to be taken to hospital.

Fracture of the Upper Arm

Fractures of the long bone (humerus) in the upper arm occur most commonly as a result of a fall, although they can occasionally result from a direct blow. There will commonly be extreme pain accompanied by bruising and/or swelling at the site of the fracture. As with other arm injuries, hospital treatment is called for but first:

1 Seat the patient.
2 Apply a sling and broad fold bandage (*see* p.63-66).

Fractures around the Elbow

These are fairly common and are characterised by pain and swelling, which will be worsened by movement. With this type of fracture, there is increased danger of damage to surrounding nerves and blood vessels, and therefore it is best to call an ambulance rather than attempt to take the patient to hospital on your own. If the elbow can still be bent, then use a sling (*see* page 65) as previously described for other arm injuries. If the arm cannot be bent:

1 Immobilise the arm by placing some padding between the arm and the trunk, then securing the arm against the body with large, broad bandages.
2 Check the patient's wrist pulse every 10 minutes. If pulse is absent loosen the bandaging and ask the patient to reposition his arm if possible until pulse returns.
3 Call an ambulance.

Fractures of the Hip and Leg

When attending a casualty with a fracture of the leg or hip it is important that an ambulance is summoned as soon as possible. The casualty should not be moved unless medical assistance cannot be summoned or you have to remove him or her from a situation of potential danger. Fractures of the hip and thigh bone are often characterised by shortening and outward rotation of the injured limb. Should you need to move the patient:

1 Gently lay the casualty on his back, supporting the injured limb with your hand, and make him as comfortable as possible.
2 Place plenty of soft padding between the legs, from the groin to the ankle. If long, straight boards or branches are available then prepare to use these as splints. One splint should be long enough to reach from the groin to the ankle and the other from the armpit to the ankle. Pad the shorter splint, lay it carefully between the legs and gently bring the sound limb alongside the fractured leg.

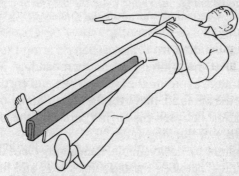

one splint should be long enough to reach from the groin to the ankle and the other from the armpit to the ankle

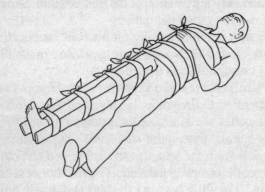

*pad and bandage the splint, avoiding the fracture site,
and tie knots over the splint*

3 Place padding from the casualty's armpit to the
ankle of the injured leg and then bandage as illustrated, avoiding the fracture site and ensuring
that the knots are tied over the splint. Apply more
padding between his or her arm and the outer
surface of the long splint.
4 If splints are not available, then gently place thick
padding between the casualty's legs and bandage the legs together, avoiding the fracture site
and ensuring that knots are tied over the pad-

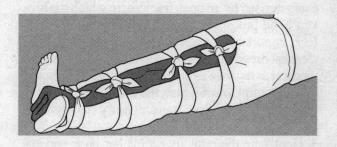

if splints are not available, then place thick padding between the casualty's legs and bandage them together, avoiding the fracture site

ding. Minimise movement and discomfort by using a thin stick to push the bandages underneath the legs.

6 Once the limbs are immobilised, if possible raise them a little to reduce the swelling. Check the ankles for signs of a pulse and the toes for numbness; loosen the bandages a little if necessary.

7 Observe the casualty for shock (*see* p.100) and ensure that he or she is kept warm and as comfortable as possible.

Fractures of the Lower Leg

Fractures to the bones of the lower leg are frequently characterised by an open fracture, in which the broken bone protrudes through the skin. It is, therefore, important to cover the wound gently with the cleanest dressing or material available and summon medical assistance as soon as possible. You should never attempt to straighten the fractured bone or to move the injured limb unnecessarily. To immobilise the leg you should:

1 Gently lie the casualty on his her back and ensure that he or she is as comfortable as possible.

2 Use two splints that both extend from well above the knee to below the ankle. Place the splints along the inner and outer side of the fractured leg, applying padding in between the splints and the leg on both sides.

3 Tie the splints to the leg with bandages or mate-

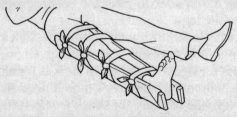

*tie the splints in up to four places, always
avoiding the site of the fracture*

rial in up to four places, always avoiding the site of the fracture. Ensure that the knots are tied over the splint.

4 If splints are not available, gently try to straighten the knee of the injured leg if it is bent. Place padding between the legs and move the sound leg alongside the injured limb.

5 Tie the feet, using a bandage tied in a figure of eight round the ankles and feet and then tie a bandage around the knee. Apply two or three more bandages, avoiding the fracture site and ensuring that the knots are tied on the uninjured side.

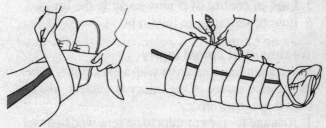

tie the feet using a figure-of-eight bandage

Fracture of the Spine

Suspected fracture of the spine should always be treated as a serious injury and medical help should be sought urgently. Fracture to the vertebrae, the small bones that make up the spine, may be complicated by the risk of damage to the spinal cord, which is enclosed within the spinal column. The spinal cord is composed of nerve tissue that transmits impulses from the brain that control many of the functions of the body. Any damage to the spinal cord could, thus, result in temporary or permanent paralysis in parts of the body, depending on where the injury occurs. It is therefore essential that the casualty is immobilised as far as possible to minimise the risk of damage.

Symptoms of spinal injury
1 The victim may complain of severe pain in the back.
2 Lack of control over movement in the limbs.
3 Loss of sensation in the limbs.

Treatment of spinal injury
When attending a casualty with a back injury, when the precise nature of the injury is unclear, **always** treat it as a fracture.
1 Arrange for the casualty to be removed to hospital, by ambulance, as soon as possible.
2 Support the casualty by gently steadying the head with your hand and placing rolled-up clothing, blankets and towels around the trunk of the body. Secure these in place with bricks, stones or heavy bags. Cover the casualty with a blanket and keep him or her as comfortable as possible.

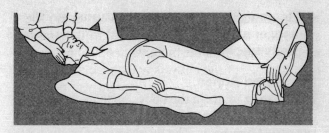

*support the casualty by gently steadying his head with
your hand and placing blankets around the trunk of
his body. Secure these in place with heavy objects*

3 If the victim is in imminent danger and has to be
moved immediately, then he or she must be supported at the head and neck, the shoulders, the
waist and the legs to ensure that the head, neck
and torso are in alignment.

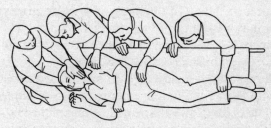

*if the victim must be moved he must be supported
so that the head, neck, shoulders, waist and legs
are in alignment*

4 The casualty should always be carried any distance on a rigid stretcher or board with the limbs gently supported.

Dislocated Bones

Articulating joints in the body , such as the shoulder or hip, are held together by strong strips of tissue called ligaments. The ligaments generally hold the joint in the correct position and ensure its correct movement, but occasionally violent movement or injury can tear the ligament, thus permitting dislocation or displacement of the bone. Contrary to popular belief, **no attempt** should be made to replace the joint, as this can result in further injury. The best course of action is to treat the dislocation as a fracture and ensure the swift removal of the patient to hospital for treatment.

Bandages and Slings

A large basic triangular bandage can be adapted for use as a sling or for folding as a broad or narrow bandage or a ring pad. These can be made by cutting a piece of material (approximately 1 metre by 1 metre) in half diagonally.

Broad bandage
Broad bandages can be used for immobilising limbs before transporting a casualty.

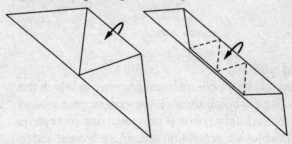

broad bandage

Using the triangular bandage, fold in the point towards the base of the bandage and then fold in half again.

Narrow bandage

A narrow bandage can be used for securing a dressing in place, making a ring pad and for fixing a figure-of-eight bandage.

Using a triangular bandage, make a broad bandage as shown above and then simply fold in half again.

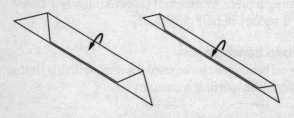

narrow bandage

Ring pad

When used on a complicated fracture, in which the bone is protruding through the skin or on a wound in which a foreign body is present, a ring pad can be used to provide protection around the wound and to prevent dressings from creating too much pressure.

1 Make a narrow bandage as shown above and wrap it once around the fingers of one hand to make a loop.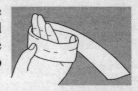

2 Take hold of the other end of the bandage and wind it around the loop, pulling it tight.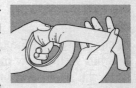

3 Continue to wind the bandage firmly around the loop until the bandage has been usedup, then tuck in the end.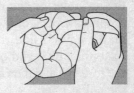

Arm sling

An arm sling should provide support for the forearm, elbow and wrist. It should be applied so that the hand is slightly higher than the elbow and the fingertips are exposed. Always apply a sling with the casualty standing or sitting down and work from the injured side to provide more support.

1 Support the arm across the chest, ensuring that the hand is slightly higher than the elbow. Take a triangular bandage and slide the base under-

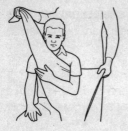

Support the arm across the chest, ensuring that the hand is slightly higher than the elbow

neath the forearm until the point of the bandage reaches well below the elbow.

2 Take the upper end of the sling, place it around the shoulder on the uninjured side, then take it around the back of the neck and then to the front on the injured side.

3 Take the lower end of the sling and fold it over the forearm and then tie it off in the hollow above the collar bone.

4 Take the point of the bandage and fold it forward

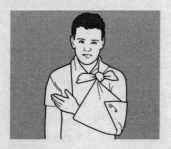

take the point of the bandage and fold it forward onto the front

onto the front, fixing it with a safety pin and ensuring that the casualty's fingertips are not covered.

Elevation sling

An elevation sling should be used to support an injury to the shoulder or when a hand wound is bleeding. The aim is to raise and support the forearm and the hand.

1 Gently place the forearm on the injured side across the chest so that the fingertips are level with the opposite shoulder. Ask the casualty to support the limb if possible.

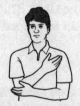

place the forearm across the chest so that fingertips are level with the opposite shoulder

2 Place the base of a triangular bandage over the raised forearm and hand so that the upper end sits on the shoulder on the uninjured side and the point reaches beyond the tip of the elbow.

3 Gently slide the base of the bandage underneath the elbow, forearm and hand.

4 Take the lower end of the sling and place it around the casualty's back and across to the

shoulder on the uninjured side. Tie it off in the hollow of the collar bone and adjust if necessary.

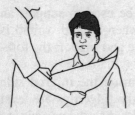

tuck the point of the sling between the forearm and the front of the sling

5 Take the point of the sling and tuck it between the forearm and the front of the sling. This will leave a fold of material that can be pinned back against the arm.

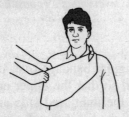

slide the base of the bandage underneath the elbow, forearm and hand

Remember – when applying bandages and slings ensure that the casualty's circulation is not affected. If it is then adjust the bandage or reposition the sling until circulation has improved.

Heart Attack and Cardiac Arrest

A heart attack is said to have occurred when a clot of blood suddenly blocks a coronary artery, one of the main blood vessels to the heart muscle, the **myocardium**. When this happens, the affected part of muscle will die because of the resulting lack of oxygen, causing the patient severe, gripping chest pain. Sometimes, the patient may have a history of **angina pectoris**, a condition in which the coronary arteries are narrowed because of the build-up of fatty deposits on the inside walls. This restricts the blood flow to the myocardium and causes severe crushing pain in the chest, not unlike that of a heart attack. It is sometimes, therefore, very difficult to distinguish between an attack of angina and a heart attack. Unlike a heart attack, angina is usually relieved by rest or by placing a tablet of glyceryl trinitrate (GTN) under the patient's tongue.

Signs and Symptoms of Heart Attack

1 Severe crushing chest pain, possibly radiating
   down one or both arms, or up into the jaw. The
   pain will not be relieved by rest or the administration of GTN.
2 Facial pallor or 'ashen' appearance, sometimes
   with blueish colouring of the lips.
3 The skin may be cold and clammy to the touch
   and the casualty may be sweating profusely.
4 The patient may suffer from breathlessness,
   weakness and dizziness.
5 Nausea and vomiting may be present.
6 The pulse may be irregular and either slow or
   fast.
7 The patient may appear profoundly anxious.
8 The patient may collapse suddenly, possibly
   without warning.

Treatment of a heart attack

1 Keep the casualty as calm and as comfortable as
   possible. Loosen any tight clothing and place
   pillows behind the head and knees to support him
   or her in a half-sitting position.
2 Phone 999 for an ambulance (or ask somebody
   to do this for you so that you can remain with
   the casualty). Be prepared to resuscitate.
3 If ordinary aspirin tablets are available, give the

casualty one and ask him or her to chew and swallow it. Recent research has shown that aspirin given immediately after the onset of heart attack can improve the victim's chances of recovery, perhaps by inhibiting further clotting in the coronary arteries.

Cardiac Arrest

Cardiac arrest is the term used to describe any sudden cessation of the heart, characterised by absence of pulse and breathing. Cardiac arrest may be the result of severe heart attack, anaphylactic shock (*see* p.99), electric shock, poisoning (including drug overdose), hypothermia or suffocation.

During cardiac arrest, the brain and heart muscle are completely starved of oxygen, a state that can be tolerated for only a few minutes before permanent damage results. **It is vital, therefore that resuscitation procedures are instigated immediately**.

The ABC of Resuscitation

Resuscitation is the emergency action required when there is sustained interruption of the oxygen supply to the brain. In order that this vital oxygen supply may be restored, three vital conditions must be met:

A The **airway** must be clear in order to permit oxy-gen-rich air to enter the lungs.

B There must be adequate **breathing** taking place in order that the oxygen can enter the blood-stream.

C The blood must be pumped around the body providing effective **circulation** to the brain and all body tissues.

When presented with an unconscious casualty, it is important to assess his or her condition **quickly** before attempting resuscitation. It is therefore important to ask the following questions:

1 Is the patient unconscious with no evidence of pulse or breathing? If so: dial 999 for an ambulance and carry out artificial ventilation and chest compression until the ambulance arrives.

2 Is the patient unconscious and not breathing but with the pulse still present? If so: give 10 breaths of artificial respiration and dial 999 for an ambulance. Continue artificial respiration until the ambulance arrives or spontaneous breathing is resumed. Check the pulse frequently.

3 Is the patient unconscious but breathing with pulse present? If so: treat any obvious injuries, dial 999 for an ambulance and place the patient in the recovery position (*see* p.83).

Always proceed by following the ABC of Resuscitation:

A *Open the airway*
1 Remove any visible obstructions from the mouth.
2 Placing two fingers under the casualty's chin, gently raise the jaw. Simultaneously, tilt the casualty's head well back by applying pressure to the forehead with your other hand.

Sometimes the airway may be blocked by the tongue as a result of loss of muscular control during unconsciousness, and this manoeuvre will lift the tongue clear.

B *Check for breathing*
Place your face close to the casualty's mouth and listen and feel for breathing for a full five seconds. At the same time look along the chest and abdomen for signs of movement.

C *Check the circulation*
If the heart is beating adequately, it will be possible to feel a **pulse** in the neck where the main carotid arteries pass on either side of the larynx on the way to the head. With the patient's head tilted back, slide your fingers between the Adam's apple

and the strap muscle and feel for the carotid pulse for five seconds.

If pulse and breathing are absent, you will need to commence artificial ventilation and chest compression immediately.

Mouth-to-Mouth or Artificial Ventilation

If the casualty is not breathing (*see* p.36), but still has a pulse, then by breathing the exhaled air from your lungs into his or hers you may be able to keep them adequately ventilated until help arrives.

1 Place the casualty flat on the back, and tilt the head back to open the airway unless you suspect spinal injury (*see* p.59) in which case lift the chin. Remove any obvious obstructions from the mouth. (Broken or loose dentures should be removed, but well-fitting dentures should remain in place).

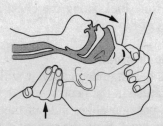

tilt the head back to open the airway

2 Pinch the nose between the index finger and thumb. Take a deep breath, then form a seal around the casualty's mouth with your own.

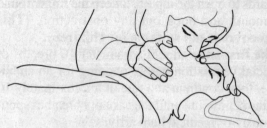

*form a seal around the casualty's
mouth with your own*

3 Blow steadily into the mouth until the chest rises. Each full inflation should take about two seconds.
4 Remove your lips from the casualty's and allow the chest to 'exhale' fully before giving a subsequent breath.

If the chest fails to rise:

1 Check that the head is tilted back correctly (*see* p.74).
2 Ensure that your lips are forming a proper seal around the patient's mouth.
3 Check that air is not escaping from the nostrils.
4 Check that the airway is not blocked by vomit or blood.

If an airway obstruction is suspected, then finger sweeps may be performed **on an adult**:

Grasp the tongue and lower jaw and pull gently upwards to open the mouth. Sweep the finger round the mouth and hook out any obstruction. (**This manoeuvre is not suitable for children**).

The first-aider should administer 10 breaths of artificial ventilation before phoning for an ambulance, then continue at a rate of approximately 10 breaths per minute until the casualty breathes spontaneously or medical help arrives.

Chest Compression

If the patient has no palpable carotid pulse and no breathing is present, then it is vital that you perform artificial ventilation and external chest compression to prevent brain damage, which is likely to occur in just a few minutes. Artificial respiration and external chest compression are together known as **cardiopulmonary resuscitation** or **CPR**.

1 Lie the patient flat on the back and feel for the point at which the lower ribs meet in the centre (the *xiphisternum)* as illustrated below.

2 Place the index and middle fingers of your left hand over this point and the heel of your right hand on the breastbone or sternum above your fingers.

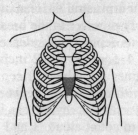

*feel for the point at which the lower ribs
meet in the centre*

3 Place your left hand directly on top of your right
hand, interlocking the fingers. Pull the fingers
away so that the heel of your right hand is the
only part in direct contact with the breastbone.

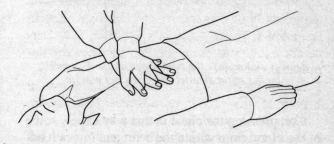

*the heel of your right hand should be the only part in
direct contact with the breastbone*

4 Keeping your arms straight, lean over the casualty and apply pressure to the breastbone. The intention is to depress and release the breastbone about 4–5cm or 1^1/$_2$–2 inches approximately 80 times per minute. Keep your hands in contact with the patient between compressions so that a smooth rhythm can be achieved. It may help to count aloud '1 and 2 and 3 and 4,' etc.

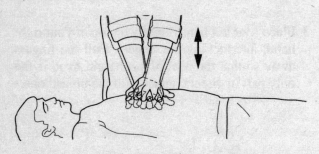

depress and release the breastbone about 4–5cm/1^1/$_2$ inches approximately 80 times per minute

Compressing the chest in this way expels some of the blood from within the heart and forces it out into the tissues and around the body. As the pressure is released, more blood will be 'sucked' into the heart to replace that expelled.

The Sequence of CPR

The most effective sequence of CPR which can be performed by one person is 15 chest compressions followed by 2 breaths of artificial respiration. If two first-aiders are present the ratio should be 5 to 1.

Do not cease CPR unless:

1 The ambulance has arrived and paramedics take over.
2 The casualty moves or begins to groan, or his or her colour improves. If this occurs, then check immediately for a carotid pulse. If the pulse has returned, and the casualty is also breathing, place him or her in the recovery position (*see* p.83) until help arrives. If the pulse has restarted but breathing has not, then continue with artificial ventilation alone at a rate of 10 breaths per minute. Check the pulse at the end of every 10 ventilations, as you will need to restart full CPR again if it stops.
3 You are exhausted and cannot continue.

CPR for Children

Although it is rare for a child to suffer a cardiac arrest, it does occasionally happen, and the first-aider should be aware that the main difference between treating a child and an adult is that the child will need to be given artificial ventilation for a full minute before dialling 999 for an ambulance. CPR can be performed on older children in much the same way as for adults, using a lighter and slightly faster technique, but must be modified as follows for use on children and babies.

1 **Airway**: gently lift the chin and tilt the head to open the airway. **Do not perform finger sweeps or touch the back of the child's throat**. Any obvious food particles or other obstruction should be gently removed from the mouth.

2 **Breathing**: look, feel and listen carefully for breathing. If it is absent, then begin artificial ventilation. This should be done as for adults, with the following exceptions.

a It is more effective to form a seal with your mouth round the child's mouth and nose than mouth alone.

b The rate of artificial ventilation will need to be twice that for an adult – about 20 breaths per minute.

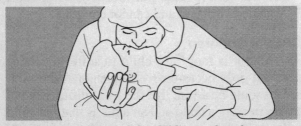

form a seal around the child's mouth and nose

c Depending on the size of the child, you will need to vary the amount of air you breathe into the lungs to make the chest rise. A baby will require only tiny puffs, whereas an older child will need more.

3 Circulation: the carotid pulse is often hard to find in an infant – if so, try the *brachial* pulse. You will find this halfway between the shoulder and the elbow on the inner side of the arm. Press lightly with your index and middle fingers (perhaps using your thumb as a brace behind the arm) for a full five seconds. If no pulse is detected, you will need to begin chest compression. Use the adult technique if the child is large, but for babies and very young children it will need to be modified as follows:

a For a **baby**, imagine a line between his or her nipples and apply chest compression with two

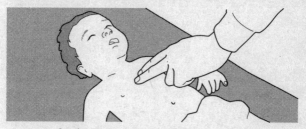

apply chest compression with two fingertips

81

fingertips just below the line. Aim to depress the chest slightly less than 1 inch or two centimetres.

b For a **toddler** or small child, identify the correct position on the chest as per the adult technique, but use the heel of one hand only. Press to a depth of 3–4 cm or $1\frac{1}{2}$ inches. In both cases, apply chest compressions at a rate of approximately 100 per minute, alternating five compressions with one breath.

Remember: if pulse and breathing are absent, artificial ventilation must be combined with chest compression. Call an ambulance as soon as possible.

The Recovery Position

An unconscious patient should always be placed in the recovery position, as the position of the head will prevent the tongue blocking the airway while allowing fluids to drain freely from the mouth. You should not leave an unconscious patient to call for help unless you have first placed him or her in the recovery position as follows:

1 Kneel beside the patient and open the airway by lifting the chin up and tilting the head. The arm nearest you should be placed at right angles to the body, with the elbow bent and the palm uppermost.

2 Bring the other arm across the patient's body and place the hand against the cheek. Hold the arm in this position.

3 With your other hand, firmly grasp the far thigh and pull the knee up and towards you. Continue pulling until the patient is on his or her side with the hand still under the cheek.

4 Adjust the hand position and tilt the head back

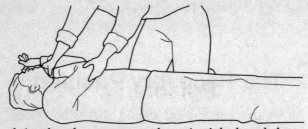

bring the other arm across the patient's body and place his hand against his cheek

again, if necessary, to ensure that the airway remains open. The hand should keep the head in the correct position.

5 The upper leg should be bent so that the hip and the knee are both at right angles.

6 Call an ambulance immediately, and make frequent checks on the patient's pulse and breathing while you wait.

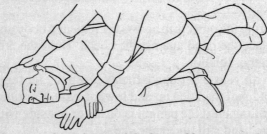

the upper leg is bent and the hip and knee are at right angles

Poisoning

By poison we mean a substance that, if it enters the body, can exert harmful effects, permanent or temporary. The routes by which a poison may enter the body are as follows:

1 **Swallowing**: may be accidental or deliberate (overdose) and includes a wide variety of substances from alcohol and illicit drugs to household cleaners or plants.
2 **Inhalation**: this can be of gases such as carbon monoxide, as well as solvents and vapours.
3 **Skin absorption**: pesticides and insecticides may be absorbed in this way, and particularly strong chemicals may also cause burns.
4 **Injection into the skin**: This includes venom, such as that injected by snakes and insects, and also illicit drugs injected by abusers.

Detailed instruction on the treatment of specific types of poisoning is outwith the scope of this book, but in general the following steps should be taken:

1 Try to obtain an accurate history of the poisoning incident. If possible, find out exactly what
the substance was, how much has been ingested
and how much time has elapsed since.
2 Obtain medical assistance immediately. **Never**
attempt to make the patient vomit as this may
cause further damage to the gastro-intestinal tract
and may even cause the patient to inhale the
vomit.
3 Place an unconscious patient in the recovery
position (*see* p.83).
4 Send specimens of the toxin to the hospital with
the patient, if possible, as well as vomit specimens. This will help in identification of the toxin
and the amount ingested.

Temperature Extremes

The body is designed to function at a temperature of between 36°C and 37.5°C (96.8°F and 99.5°F). Generally, the core temperature is kept constantly within these limits by a heat-regulating mechanism in the brain. Occasionally, the body temperature can rise or fall to a level wherein this mechanism can no longer effectively regulate the temperature, resulting in the following conditions:

Hypothermia

Hypothermia occurs when the core temperature of the body falls to below 35°C (95°F). Once below 35°C, shivering stops and the patient no longer feels cold but appears lethargic and apathetic. If the body temperature continues to drop, hypothermia sufferers may become increasingly confused and may even begin to experience sensations of heat and attempt to remove their clothing. At a temperature of below 30°C (86°F), the muscles become rigid, and uncon-

First Aid

sciousness will eventually ensue. A body temperature of less than 27°C (80.6°F) will eventually cause
cardiac arrest. Elderly people and babies are particularly susceptible to hypothermia, but young, healthy
people can also be at risk if exposed to extremely
low temperatures for lengthy periods of time.

Treatment of Hypothermia

1 Bring the patient indoors and remove any wet
   clothing.
2 If indoors, and the casualty is capable of moving
   unaided, fill a bath with hot water (40°C/104°F)
   and completely immerse him or her in it. If the
   casualty is frail or elderly, allow him or her to
   warm up gradually in bed, well covered. Avoid
   using electric blankets and hot-water bottles.
3 Give the patient something hot and sweet to drink.
   Avoid alcohol as it exacerbates hypothermia.
4 Call a doctor. If the casualty becomes unconscious,
   call an ambulance and be prepared to resuscitate.

Heat Exhaustion

Heat exhaustion usually occurs gradually and is particularly common in those who have been working
or exercising vigorously in unaccustomed heat. The
symptoms are often similar to those of shock (*see*
p.100), as a result of the excessive loss of fluids
through perspiration. The sufferer's temperature

may be normal or only slightly raised, the skin cold and clammy, and the pulse fast and weak. In addition, the loss of salt because of excessive perspiration may cause painful muscle cramps. The patient may also be hyperventilating.

Treatment of Heat Exhaustion

1 Remove the patient out of direct sunlight and heat to a shaded, cool place.
2 Ask the casualty to lie down and support his or her legs in a raised position.
3 Encourage the casualty to drink plenty of weak salty water (about one teaspoon of salt per litre of water is sufficient).
4 If the patient recovers quickly, he or she should still be encouraged to see a doctor.
5 Should the patient become unconscious, place him or her in the recovery position (*see* p.83) and call an ambulance. While you are waiting for help to arrive, keep a check on the patient's pulse and breathing.

Heatstroke

Heatstroke often occurs rapidly, resulting in unconsciousness within a few minutes, although there is sometimes a warning period when the patient may complain of feeling unwell or strange. It occurs when the brain's 'thermostat' fails as a result of prolonged exposure to high temperature in the surroundings or of illness with high fever.

Symptoms of Heatstroke

1 Dizziness, headache, discomfort, unease and confusion.
2 The skin will feel hot and dry and appear flushed.
3 The pulse will be fast and strong.
4 The patient may collapse and become unconscious.

Treatment of heatstroke

1 Remove the casualty quickly to a cool place and remove the outer clothing. Summon medical help immediately.
2 Wrap the casualty in a sheet and keep it wet until the oral temperature falls to 38°C (100.4°F).
3 When the temperature has returned to a safe level, remove the wet sheet and substitute it with a dry one. Keep a close watch on the patient, and be prepared to repeat step 2 if the temperature rises again.
4. If the casualty becomes unconscious, place him or her in the recovery position (*see* p.83) and be prepared to resuscitate. Call an ambulance immediately.

Unconsciousness

Common Causes of Unconsciousness

1 Impairment of the blood supply to the brain. This may be a result of:
   a Fainting
   b Shock
   c Cardiac arrest
2 Impairment of oxygen supply to the brain. This may result from:
   a Choking
   b Suffocation
   c Carbon monoxide poisoning
3 Direct damage to the brain, i.e. head injury.
4 Compression of the brain. This may be a result of:
   a Skull fracture
   b Infection
   c Tumour
   d Stroke

91

5 Alteration of the chemical balance of the brain's blood supply. This may be caused by:
  a Poisoning (including drugs and alcohol)
  b Low blood sugar (hypoglycaemia)
6 Other causes, such as:
  a Epilepsy
  b Abnormally high body temperature
  c Electrocution

First Aid for the Unconscious

Unconsciousness is caused by a variety of conditions THAT interrupt normal brain function. Unlike sleep, the casualty cannot be easily or completely roused in response to stimuli such as sound or pain. The first-aider should always bear in mind that there is a danger that the airway will become blocked during unconsciousness, either by vomit or by the tongue falling backwards, causing an obstruction of the airway. Therefore always follow the following steps:
1 Lift the chin and gently tilt the head to open the airway. (If the patient begins to vomit, place in the recovery position.) If you suspect that there may be spinal injury, open the airway by lifting the chin. Do not attempt to tilt the head.
2 Check the pulse and respiration. Be prepared to resuscitate if necessary.

3 Check the casualty for any heavy external bleeding or fractures and treat accordingly.

4 Place the patient in the recovery position (*see* p.83) if you are satisfied that there is no serious neck or spinal injury.

5 If full consciousness has not been regained within three minutes, telephone 999 for an ambulance.

Do Not attempt to give the unconscious patient anything by mouth.

Do Not attempt to move the patient unnecessarily, or to make him or her sit up.

Head Injuries and Loss of Consciousness

The brain is encased within the hard bony skull and cushioned by cerebro-spinal fluid to protect it from injury. It transmits impulses via the spinal chord, which runs down the neck and spine, to all the nerves of the body. The brain and spinal chord are extremely fragile and incapable of repairing themselves, hence the protection of the skull and spine.

Fracture of the Skull

Although skull fracture is frequently indicative of a potentially serious and life-threatening condition, be aware that the real danger is damage to the brain itself. There may be fragments of bony skull causing pressure or compression on the brain (depressed fracture) and the resulting indentation of the skull may be missed as a result of swelling in the scalp. Therefore all injuries to the head should be treated with the utmost caution and suspicion, especially if any of the following signs of cerebral compression are present:

1 Vomiting, persistent headache or yawning.
2 Brief or partial loss of consciousness, or full unconsciousness.
3 Pupils of unequal sizes, which may enlarge and fail to constrict in response to light if compression increases.
4 One-sided paralysis or weakness of the face or body.
5 Irregular or noisy breathing, becoming increasingly slower.
6 Slow, strong pulse.
7 High temperature and flushed face.
8 Leakage of watery blood or straw-coloured fluid from the nose or ear.

Remember that an injury above chest level should be treated as a suspected spinal injury. In all cases, call 999 for an ambulance and treat as for unconsciousness while awaiting its arrival.

Diabetic Coma

Normally, an organ called the pancreas produces

a hormone called insulin that regulates the level of sugar in our blood. In diabetes mellitus, the pancreas fails to perform this role adequately. Sufferers may display symptoms such as tiredness, loss of weight, severe thirst, and the passing of large quantities of urine. Once diagnosed, patients can lead a relatively normal life with a few modifications. Mild diabetes may be controlled simply by restricting intake of carbohydrates in the diet, or by taking oral medication. More severe forms, however, will need to be controlled by regular injections of insulin and careful monitoring of energy intake.

Diabetic Emergencies – Hypoglycaemia and Hyperglycaemia

If the blood sugar level falls below normal, then a condition known as hypoglycaemia is said to exist. Without adequate levels of sugar in the blood, the brain can no longer function normally. Most diabetics are aware of the steps they must take to prevent this occurring, and can usually identify the first symptoms of an attack and take the appropriate action – normally the ingestion of sugar or glucose tablets. However, if an attack becomes advanced, unconsciousness will eventually occur and failure to act quickly can result in brain damage.

How to Recognise a Hypoglycaemic Attack

1 The attack will usually be rapid in onset. The patient may complain of weakness, tiredness, hunger or feeling faint. Ask if he or she is diabetic, or look for a Medic-alert bracelet or warning card.
2 The patient may experience palpitations and muscle tremors.
3 If no sugar is taken, the patient may become confused or aggressive.
4 The skin will become cold, clammy and sweaty.
5 Breathing may become shallow.
6 The patient may eventually become unconscious.

Treatment of Hypoglycaemia

1 Aim to raise the blood sugar levels as quickly as possible by giving the victim sugary food or drink. Ascertain whether or not the patient carries a supply of glucagon for injection for such emergencies, in which case follow the instructions enclosed. If there is no improvement within five minutes or . . .
2 . . . if the victim is unconscious, place him or her in the recovery position and be prepared to resuscitate.
3 Call for an ambulance.

Hyperglycaemia

In hyperglycaemia, the pancreas fails to produce enough insulin to prevent excessive levels of sugar in the blood. Once diagnosed, diabetics will be able to prevent hyperglycaemia by balancing their dietary intake of sugar and by regular insulin injections.

Occasionally, hyperglycaemia can cause unconsciousness, but the condition generally develops gradually over a period of days or weeks. The symptoms of hyperglycaemic coma are as follows:

1 Dry skin
2 Faint smell of acetone (similar to nail varnish remover or mown grass) on the breath
3 Rapid pulse
4 Deep, laboured breathing.

Dial 999 for an ambulance or transport the patient to hospital immediately for treatment.

Shock and Allergic Reactions

An allergy is an abnormal response by the body to a specific stimulus or allergen. These can be familiar, everyday substances such as house dust, pollen or animal fur, causing mild symptoms such as sneezing, itchiness or a rash. Hay fever, for instance, is an allergic response to pollens in the air and is most commonly experienced in the summer months. Similarly, many people may suffer unpleasant allergic reactions after ingesting particular foods. Shellfish, nuts and eggs are often the culprits, and most sufferers quickly manage to identify those foods that cause the reaction and thereafter avoid them. Sometimes, patients can also experience an allergic response to some drugs, such as penicillin, and medical practitioners will always bear this in mind when prescribing medication.

Although allergies can be extremely unpleasant and distressing for the sufferer, they will rarely necessitate first aid or emergency treatment. However, a patient may occasionally experience a severe and life-threatening reaction to an allergen. This is known as anaphylactic shock and requires urgent medical attention. This reaction can occur in response to bee or wasp stings or the ingestion of nuts or any food that causes allergy in the sufferer and can therefore be extremely difficult to diagnose.

Anaphylactic Shock

1 Does the patient's skin have a rash or red blotches (hives)?
2 Is there any swelling on any part of the patient's body, but particularly on the face, the lips or the tongue?
3 Is he or she having difficulty in breathing? This may indicate swelling in the airway.
4 Is he or she experiencing tightness in his chest?
5 Is the skin colour normal or does it appear greyish or even blue?
6 Is the patient unconscious or suffering from seizures?
7 Can the pulse be felt? Is it weak or rapid?

Any of the above symptoms can develop within a few moments of the initial exposure to the allergen. The treatment for severe anaphylactic shock is the administration of the drug adrenaline and of oxygen. Increasingly, allergy sufferers identified as being at risk of anaphylactic shock will be issued with pre-packed injections of adrenaline that are quick and simple to use, so it is sensible to check whether or not your patient is thus equipped. Otherwise, there is no specific treatment other than remaining with your patient until medical help arrives. He or she should be kept in a comfortable upright position to assist breathing, unless he or she loses consciousness, in which case the recovery position is preferred.

Shock

When referred to in medical emergency, shock is taken to signify a life-threatening condition caused by the failure of the circulatory system to pump blood around the body. Internal and external bleeding can cause this, as can heart attack, anaphylactic shock and excessive loss of body fluids such as occurs in diarrhoea or severe burns. The body tries to maximise the use of remaining body fluids by withdrawing them from the surface and extremities of the body to the centre. This can progressively produce the following symptoms:

1 The patient's skin becomes cold, grey and

clammy as the body attempts to divert blood supplies to the vital organs.

2 The pulse becomes rapid as the heart works harder to circulate the reduced volume of blood.

3 The pulse becomes weaker and may become irregular as the blood volume and pressure fall.

4 The patient becomes weak and giddy as oxygen fails to reach the muscles and brain.

5 The patient's breathing becomes rapid and shallow, and he may appear to be attempting to yawn or gulp in air ('air hunger').

6 The patient may complain of nausea and actually vomit.

7 The patient may experience thirst as the brain senses that the body needs to make up a shortfall in fluid.

8 The patient may become restless and agitated as the oxygen supply to the brain deteriorates.

9 The patient will lose consciousness, and the pulse at the wrist may become unpalpable.

10 The heart will stop.

It is vital to identify and treat the causes of shock immediately.

Always summon medical help at the earliest possible opportunity, but it may be possible to slow the progression of shock by taking prompt action to stop bleeding from an open wound.

A-Z of Illnesses and Disorders and Quick Guide to Symptoms

Symptoms and Self-Diagnosis: A Word of Warning

This list of conditions and symptoms is **not** comprehensive. It is included in this guide to *First Aid* as an aid to recognising those conditions and illnesses that need immediate first aid or medical attention and have symptoms that are of sudden onset, or are caused by a recent trauma, injury or infection.

From even a brief study of the contents of this section, it will be apparent that most illnesses and disorders produce a range of symptoms. For any given illness or condition, certain symptoms may be more pronounced in one individual than in another. Diagnosis is a skilled undertaking, which must always be carried out by a doctor and not deduced from the pages of a book. Also, it is overwhelmingly the case that early diagnosis and treatment produce the best results and outlook for the patient.

If you are experiencing any symptoms, however slight, that are causing you concern, you should *always* consult a doctor. **Do not** attempt to diagnose and treat yourself.

Given the variable nature of the symptoms of many illnesses and disorders, the latter may be listed under more than one heading in the Quick Reference to Symptoms on page 107.

Quick Reference
to Symptoms

Please note: This list of conditions and symptoms is **not** comprehensive. It is included as an aid to recognising those conditions and illnesses that need immediate first aid or medical attention and have symptoms that are of sudden onset, or are caused by a recent trauma, injury or infection.

HEAD AND NECK

headache that may be accompanied by other symptoms, e.g. numbness or weakness, nausea and vomiting, confusion, vision disturbance

Possible cause:

dizziness, loss of balance, fainting, convulsions, paralysis and loss of consciousness *see* **General Symptoms**

eyes and eyelids – inflammation, itching, pain, discharge, swelling, protrusion

Possible cause:
corneal foreign bodies   153

eyes – visual disturbance, loss of vision

Possible cause:
head injury   180
migraine   199
retinal detachment   220
stroke   226
thromboembolism   232
transient ischaemic attack   238

eyes – sensitivity to light

Possible cause:
meningitis   197
migraine   199

ears – discharge, pain, ringing noise, nausea, vomiting, deafness, dizziness

Possible cause:
ruptured eardrum   223

mouth – soreness, ulceration, dryness, bleeding

Possible cause:
botulism   139

mouth – paralysis or difficulty with speech

Possible cause:
stroke   226

neck – sudden, spontaneous stiffness

Possible cause:

throat – soreness, coughing, hoarseness

Possible cause:

CHEST

chest pain

Possible cause:

chest pain with other symptoms, e.g. breathing difficulty, cough, fever, chills

Possible cause:

breathlessness, wheezing, difficulty in breathing, cyanosis (blue tinge to the skin), anxiety *see also* **chest pain with other symptoms**

Possible cause:

ABDOMEN

abdominal pain, sudden or severe

Possible cause:

gastrointestinal symptoms – diarrhoea, nausea, vomiting, abdominal swelling, abdominal pain, indigestion, constipation, abnormal faeces

Possible cause:

BACK, LIMBS AND JOINTS AND MUSCLES

back – lower back pain, sudden or severe
Possible cause:

prolapsed intervertebral disc	212
sciatica	224

joints and limbs – pain with general stiffness and weakness and other symptoms such as swelling, inflammation and pain
Possible cause:

anaphylactic shock	123
bone fracture	137
dislocation	158

leg – pain and tenderness
Possible cause:

thromboembolism	232
thrombosis	233

general muscular weakness, twitches or spasms – abnormal and involuntary
Possible cause:

convulsions	151
epilepsy	168

RECTUM AND ANUS

rectum – bleeding, pain and blood in faeces
Possible cause:

dysentery	161

REPRODUCTIVE SYSTEM

vagina – abnormal bleeding from

Possible cause:

testicles – swelling and pain

Possible cause:

SKIN

skin – rash with accompanying symptoms of fever, aches and pains, and chills

Possible cause:

PSYCHOLOGICAL DISTURBANCE

behavioural changes – confusion, loss of memory, abnormal fatigue, aggression, etc

Possible cause:

GENERAL SYMPTOMS

sudden fever, fatigue and weakness, dizziness, chills, aches and pains, with possible other symptoms, e.g. fainting, rapid pulse, vomiting and nausea

loss of balance, dizziness, fainting, convulsions, paralysis and loss of consciousness

bleeding or bruising – spontaneous or abnormal

A-Z of Illnesses and Disorders

abruptio placentae

Description: bleeding from the placenta after the 28th week of pregnancy, which may result in the placenta becoming completely or partially separated from the wall of the uterus (womb).

Persons affected: females during pregnancy.

Organ or part of body involved: uterus.

Symptoms and indications: these depend upon the degree of separation of the placenta and so range from slight to severe but include bleeding from the vagina, pain in the abdomen and abdominal hardness. In very serious untreated cases: maternal shock and foetal distress with possible fatal outcome for both mother and baby.

Always tell your doctor if you experience bleeding at any time during pregnancy.

Treatment: Admittance to hospital for rest and observation. An ultrasound examination is usually carried out to establish the diagnosis of abruptio placentae as the symptoms are very similar to those of

PLACENTA PRAEVIA . If the bleeding is slight, the foetus is in good health and the pregnancy is not near to term, butcontinued bed rest is required until the bleeding stops. If the bleeding worsens, delivery of the foetus by Caesarian section is usually required. (Delivery may sometimes be vaginal if labour has already started.)

Causes and risk factors: the cause is unknown, but abruptio placentae is more likely to occur in women who already have children, who are aged over 35 and who smoke. Also it may result from an accidental blow in the abdominal region.

adult respiratory distress syndrome (ARDS)

Description: severe respiratory failure, which is often fatal, brought about by a number of different disorders. In newborn babies, a similar condition is known as hyaline membrane disease.

Persons most commonly affected: adults and children (except newborn) of both sexes and all ages.

Symptoms and indications: a lack of oxygen in the blood, which is indicated by a blueness (cyanosis) of the skin, an abnormally rapid rate of breathing (tachypnoea) and a raised heartbeat rate (tachycardia). There is pulmonary oedema (a collection of fluid in the lungs) and the substance known as surfactant, which prevents the lungs' sacs (alveoli) from collapsing and allows oxygen to pass in and carbon dioxide to pass out, is lost. These conditions lead to the lungs becoming stiff and ineffective; death follows without emergency medical intervention. A person with signs of this disorder requires urgent medical treatment.

Treatment: intensive care treatment, including mechanical ventilation of the lungs and management of the patient's fluid balance to reduce pulmonary oedema. Also, the underlying cause of the respiratory failure is treated if this is possible. Surfactant may be given by means of a nebuliser or aerosol.

Causes and risk factors: there are a variety of different causes of this disorder, which may be broadly divided into five categories:

- Physical causes, including injury to the lungs, inhalation of water as in drowning, vomit or other foreign substance.
- Bacterial, viral or fungal infection of the lungs or other part of the body, as in various diseases including pneumonia, sepsis, poliomyelitis.
- As a response by the patient's immune system following blood transfusion or cardiopulmonary bypass surgery.
- Accidental inhalation of poisonous fumes and smoke, ingestion of certain chemicals and drugs.
- As a complication of various other diseases and

disorders, including asthma, emphysema, muscular dystrophy, pancreatitis, Guillain-Barré syndrome, uraemia, myasthenia gravis.

Patients who receive mechanical ventilation for a long period may develop complications in the form of secondary infections and pneumothorax, which require additional treatment. The survival rate for patients with this condition is about 50per cent, and those who respond well suffer little lung damage. There is a greater likelihood of lung damage in those patients needing prolonged mechanical ventilation.

alcohol poisoning *see also* pages 85–86
Description: a single episode of severe overconsumption of alcohol is usually accidental and can result in alcohol poisoning, unconsciousness and even death. Alcohol depresses the central nervous system. As the concentration of alcohol in the blood increases, motor functions are impaired. With continued and excessive consumption, especially in those who are unused to alcohol, motor functions and coordination will eventually become severely disturbed and lead to unconsciousness and with risk to life.
Persons most commonly affected: both sexes and all age groups after adolescence, although more common in males.

Organ or part of body involved: brain, liver, heart.
Symptoms and indications: the casualty's breath will smell of alcohol, he or she may be vomiting and they may be partly or already unconscious. If unconscious, the casualty will be breathing deeply and the face will be moist and flushed. In the early stages of unconsciousness the pulse will be strong and fast, in the later stages the breathing becomes very shallow, the pulse is still rapid but weak, the face will look bloated and the eyes will be blood-shot with the pupils dilated.
Treatment: if you suspect that someone is suffering from alcoholic poisoning, ensure that the person has an open airway. If the person becomes unconscious, has vomited or you think that he or she is likely to vomit, place the person in the recovery position and obtain medical assistance immediately.
Causes and risk factors: personality and the environment in which a person lives (e.g. a young person in a family or social group in which alcohol is important) and stress related to work and family and personal relationships are all significant factors.

allergy

Description: a state of hypersensitivity (or heightened or oversensitivity) in an affected individual to a particular substance, called the 'allergen'. This produces a characteristic response whenever the person is exposed to the allergen.

Persons most commonly affected: both sexes and all age groups.

Organ or part of body involved: various parts of the body, depending on the nature of the allergy, but including skin, respiratory system, joints and gastrointestinal system.

Symptoms and indications: symptoms usually develop rapidly, within a few minutes, and depend on the nature of the allergy (*see also* ANAPHYLACTIC SHOCK, ASTHMA and p. 99). Common symptoms include nettle rash and skin reactions, swellings and puffiness, e.g. around eyes, wheezing and breathing difficulties (*see also* pages 21–23), HEADACHES, stomach pains, sickness and diarrhoea. Medical advice should be sought.

Treatment: this depends upon the nature of the reaction but commonly involves the taking of antihistamine drugs. If the allergic response is more serious, as in an asthma attack, hospital treatment may be required, with the administration of bronchodilator and corticosteroid drugs by inhalation. If the allergic response is in the rare form of prompt emergency treatment is necessary with the administration of adrenaline by means of an injection.

This condition is fatal unless emergency treatment is promptly received.

Causes and risk factors: in a nonallergic, unaffected person, antibodies present in the bloodstream destroy their particular allergens (antigens). However, in an allergic, affected person this reaction causes some cell damage and there is a release of substances such as histamine and bradykinin, which cause the reaction. Many substances, usually of a protein nature, can be allergens. The list includes many common foods, such as eggs, strawberries and shellfish, colourings and additives used in foods, plants and pollen, mites or dust from animals such as cats, dogs, horses and the feathers of birds. If the allergen is known then it may be possible for the individual to avoid exposure to it. Sometimes it is possible to decrease sensitivity to a particular allergen by gradually increasing exposure under careful medical supervision. However, a person may be allergic to a range of substances. In many people there may be a genetic element, with a family history of allergy.

altitude sickness

Description: also known as mountain sickness, this condition affects individuals (usually mountaineers) who are exposed to high altitudes to which they are unaccustomed.

Persons most commonly affected: both sexes and all age groups (normally adults).

Organ or part of body involved: lungs, respiratory system, blood, brain.

Symptoms and indications: rapid, deep breathing (hyperventilation), nausea, headache, exhaustion, anxiety. In severe cases, there may be breathing difficulties as aresult of pulmonary oedema caused by fluid collecting in the lungs. This is a dangerous condition that may prove fatal.

Treatment: the person must be brought down to a lower altitude for rest and further acclimatisation. An individual with pulmonary oedema requires urgent medical treatment in hospital.

Causes and risk factors: the cause is climbing to a high altitude (above 3000 metres) too quickly without giving the body time to adjust to lower oxygen levels and reduced atmospheric pressure. This causes the person to breathe more deeply and rapidly (hyperventilate) with a consequent lowering of CO_2 levels in the blood. It is essential to allow the body to adjust by spending time at a particular altitude and attaining height gradually. Usually, the symptoms are relatively mild, but if they prove to be disabling the climber must return to a lower altitude.

anaphylactic shock *see also* pages 100–101
Description: anaphylaxis is a response exhibited by a hypersensitive (highly sensitive) person when confronted with a particular substance or antigen. It results from the release of histamine in body tissues following the antigen-antibody reaction within cells. An allergic reaction is an example of mild anaphylaxis (*see* ALLERGY). Anaphylactic shock is a much rarer and more serious condition that can follow the injection of drugs or vaccines, or a bee sting, to which the person is hypersensitive. Its onset is immediate and results from a widespread release of histamine in the body.
Persons most commonly affected: all age groups and both sexes.
Organ or part of body involved: respiratory and circulatory system, skin and heart.
Symptoms and indications: the symptoms appear rapidly in the form of severe breathing difficulties, swelling (oedema), acute itching and rash (urticaria), a fall in blood pressure leading to fainting, and loss of consciousness. Heart failure leading to shock, cardiac arrest and death. Anaphylactic shock is a medical emergency and requires immediate prompt treatment.
Treatment: the only effective treatment is an intramuscular injection of adrenaline (epinephrine) that

should be given as soon as possible. A person receiving prompt treatment usually makes a full recovery.

Causes and risk factors: there are a variety of causes for this condition, including vaccines, drugs and medications, especially if injected, wasp or bee stings and insect bites, and some foods such as peanuts, beans, shellfish, eggs and certain types of fruit. A person with a history of allergy in the form of eczema, asthma or hay fever, or who has had a previous mild reaction to a particular substance, is likely to be at greater risk.

aneurysm

Description: a balloon-like swelling of the wall of an artery that occurs when it becomes weakened or damaged in some way.

Persons most commonly affected: adult persons of both sexes, especially in older age.

Organ or part of body involved: arteries in any part but especially in the brain (circle of Willis), aorta or leg arteries.

Symptoms and indications: these vary a great deal depending on the site and size of the aneurysm. Pain may be present if the aneurysm compresses nerves, and also bulging, which may throb and contract and expand. A thoracic aneurysm may press on the windpipe and cause a hoarseness of the voice and a cough. A brain aneurysm may cause a throbbing headache and changes in the eyes (pupils of different sizes) or disturbances of vision. If the aneurysm affects the heart there may be disturbances of heartbeat rhythm and other symptoms of cardiac failure. Oedema also occurs, causing swelling of the skin because of interference with the circulation. An aneurysm is a medical emergency, and the doctor should be called immediately.

Treatment: hospital treatment and surgery to remove or isolate the aneurysm and restore the circulation by means of a graft or anastomosis (artificial joining of sections of the arteries involved). Anticoagulant drugs may be needed after surgery and penicillin if the aneurysm was caused by syphilis.

Causes and risk factors: aneurysms occur because of a weakness in the walls of the arteries, which is usually caused by atheroma or atherosclerosis (a degenerative disease of the arterial walls with scarring and a buildup of fatty deposits). Syphilis is another cause, especially affecting the aorta in the thorax. More rarely, there may be a congenital weakness affecting the arteries, especially in the case of aneurysms in the circle of Willis (a circle of arteries supplying, and sited beneath, the brain).

The danger with aneurysm is that of rupture causing haemorrhage and death, and also the risk of
stroke. Some changes in the arteries tend to occur
naturally in older people. Atheroma or atherosclerosis is more likely to be a problem in people eating a diet rich in saturated fat. Smoking, obesity,
high blood pressure and a sedentary lifestyle are
additional contributory factors.

angina pectoris
Description: a pain and feeling of choking felt in
the chest, brought on by exercise or exertion and
relieved by rest. It occurs when the blood supply
to the heart muscle is inadequate.
Persons most commonly affected: more common in
men in middle and older age; postmenopausal women.
Organ or part of body involved: coronary arteries.
Symptoms and indications: the main symptom is pain
behind the breastbone, brought on by exertion and
relieved by rest. The pain may be more or less severe and often passes to the left arm and face. There
may be a numbness or feeling of heaviness and tingling in the whole or part of the left arm. Also, there
may be a feeling of choking and breathlessness and
tightness across the chest. A person with symptoms
of angina should always seek medical advice.
Treatment: diagnosis is usually confirmed in hos-

pital by means of an electrocardiogram. Treatment involves rest and avoidance of the exertion that caused the angina attack. The patient needs to keep warm, especially in severe winter weather, and may need to adjust the diet and lose weight. Changes in lifestyle may be necessary to avoid tiredness and stress. Medication in the form of glyceryl trinitrate tablets (or amyl nitrite for inhalation) are used to bring immediate relief during an angina attack. It may be necessary for the patient to undergo coronary-artery bypass surgery or angioplasty.

Causes and risk factors: angina pectoris is caused by an inadequate blood supply to the heart muscle. During exercise, the demand for blood supplied by the coronary arteries is increased and if the supply is insufficient because the arteries are damaged, chest pain results. The most common reason for this damage is atherosclerosis or atheroma, along with spasm of the coronary arteries. Less commonly, aortic valve disease or disease in the aorta itself may be a cause of angina pectoris. Factors thought to contribute to the development of this condition include inadequate exercise, a diet rich in saturated fats and salt, high blood pressure (hypertension), stress, obesity, smoking and diabetes mellitus. Also, genetic factors, i.e. a family history of coronary-artery disease.

appendicitis (acute)

Description: the vermiform appendix is a blind-ended tube, about 9 or 10 cm long, projecting from the caecum (a pouch), which is the first part of the large intestine. Appendicitis is inflammation of the vermiform appendix, which, in its acute form, is the most common abdominal emergency in the western world.

Persons most commonly affected: all age groups and both sexes, but it is rare in young children under the age of two. It is most common in young people up to the age of 25.

Organ or part of body involved: vermiform appendix.

Symptoms and indications: the symptoms include abdominal pain that often begins over the navel and then moves to low on the right ileac fossa, with pronounced local tenderness. The pain is severe and worse with movement e.g. coughing or deep breathing, etc. Also, there may be nausea and vomiting, diarrhoea, loss of appetite and fever. Eventually, there is abdominal swelling and tenderness. A person with symptoms of appendicitis should seek immediate medical attention, as it is an emergency condition.

Treatment: usually appendicitis occurs in the acute form, requiring hospital treatment or appendicectomy – the surgical removal of the appendix. The condition is normally completely cured with prompt surgery but is dangerous if left untreated.

Causes and risk factors: blockage and subsequent infection of the appendix are the causes of appendicitis, which can occur at any time. Danger arises if the condition is left untreated or misdiagnosed. In this instance, the appendix may become the site of an abscess or may become gangrenous and rupture, causing PERITONITIS. This arises because infected material from the burst appendix spreads into the peritoneal cavity, and it is often fatal. Rupture of the appendix is more likely to occur in older patients.

asphyxia

Description: this translates literally as an absence of pulse but is used in a wider sense to describe the state of suffocation. During the course of this, breathing and heartbeat cease and oxygen fails to reach the tissues and organs. Brain cells are irreparably damaged if deprived of oxygen for more than about four minutes.

Persons most commonly affected: all age groups and both sexes.

Organ or part of body involved: lungs, heart, respiratory and circulatory systems.

Symptoms and indications: in most cases, the person fights and gasps for breath, has a rapid pulse rate, throbbing in the head as blood pressure rises and blueness of the skin. Eventually, there may be convulsions, followed by a state of paralysis, unconsciousness and death. However, in some instances, where the inhalation of toxic fumes such as carbon monoxide is responsible for the asphyxia, death may occur peacefully, without the struggles described above and during sleep. A person suffering from asphyxia requires urgent, prompt treatment if death is to be avoided.

Treatment: this depends on the cause of the asphyxia in the first instance. If the cause is choking because of a piece of food, or other foreign body, becoming lodged in the windpipe, this must be removed. A young child can be held upside down by the legs and struck firmly on the back, as this results in the object being dislodged more easily. In adults, blows on the back over the shoulder blades in time with coughing may help the object to be expelled. However, it may be necessary to perform the Heimlich's manoeuvre (*see* page 30). The person carrying out the procedure encircles the patient from behind with his or her arms. A fist is made with one hand slightly above the patient's navel and below the ribs. With the free hand, the fist is thrust firmly into the abdomen with a rapid, upward push, which may need to be repeated several times. As a result of this, the foreign body is expelled through or into the patient's mouth. In the situation outlined above, the patient usually recovers rapidly and resumes normal breathing. If toxic fumes are the cause of asphyxia, the person must be removed into clean air (*see* CARBON MONOXIDE POISONING). In all cases of asphyxia, the essential aim of treatment is to increase the amount of oxygen in the blood. If respiration and heartbeat have stopped, emergency resuscitation methods (mouth-to-mouth breathing and external cardiac massage) must be used. Once respiration and heartbeat have started (or if still present), the person requires further intensive care treatment in hospital.

Causes and risk factors: as indicated above, there are a number of different causes of asphyxia, including DROWNING, strangulation, choking and inhalation of toxic fumes. Also, swelling leading to obstruction of breathing and asphyxia may occur in certain diseases and conditions, including diphtheria, asthma, CROUP and infection of a wound.

asthma

Description: a chronic, hypersensitive condition characterised by recurrent bouts of illness or asthma attacks. The affected person has breathing difficulties caused by a narrowing of the airways (the bronchi and bronchioles) leading to the lungs.

Persons most commonly affected: all age groups except newborn babies, often beginning in early childhood. In childhood, more boys than girls suffer from asthma but in adult life both sexes are affected equally.

Organ or part of body involved: airways (bronchi and bronchioles) and lungs.

Symptoms and indications: the main symptoms are breathlessness and a wheezing cough that may be worse at night. The extent to which the bronchi are narrowed varies considerably and governs the severity of the attack. In a severe attack, the breathing rate increases considerably and is rapid and shallow. The pulse rate also increases. In a very severe attack, the person may be so breathless as to make speech impossible and may show signs of cyanosis, i.e. a bluish colour of the skin because of a lack of oxygen in the blood. A severe asthma attack or one that does not respond to the usual controlling medication taken by the patient is an emergency condition and medical help should be sought immediately. Prolonged and repeated attacks of asthma, with no break in between, are called *status asthmaticus*. This also is a serious emergency that can cause death due to exhaustion and respiratory failure.

Treatment: the day-to-day treatment of asthma is one of management to avoid the occurrence of an attack. This includes avoidance of the particular substance or allergen that triggers the asthma, if this is known and if it is possible to do so. Drugs used in the treatment of asthma are of two kinds. Bronchodilators are used to dilate the airways, and these include beta-adrenergic agonists such as salbutamol and anticholinergics such as theophyllines. The second group are anti-inflammatory drugs, which are inhaled corticosteroids and sodium cromoglycate. Most of the drugs used in the management of asthma are inhaled. Patients with severe asthma attacks or status asthmaticus require immediate admittance to hospital and treatment in intensive care.

Causes and risk factors: the cause of asthma is swelling and inflammation of the walls of the airways, and contraction of the muscles, so that the openings are narrowed. This is triggered by a hypersensitive response to a number of different allergens. Common allergens include pollen, dust from mites, domestic pets, birds and farm animals and airborne pollutants from, e.g. car exhaust emissions. An asthma sufferer may have other hypersensitive conditions such as eczema or hay fever, and there may be a genetic element with prevalence within a family. Exercise and stress may also trigger an asthma attack, and the condition is exacerbated by exposure to tobacco smoke.

atrial fibrillation

Description: a serious form of arrhythmia affecting the atria (upper chambers) of the heart.

Persons most commonly affected: adults of both sexes in middle and older age, usually with some form of heart disease or damage.

Organ or part of body involved: heart.

Symptoms and indications: irregular, rapid heartbeat and pulse, which are felt as unpleasant palpitations and may cause chest pain, breathlessness, faintness and weakness. There may be symptoms of stroke because of the formation of blood clots in the heart. In severe cases, this may lead to heart failure and death. Immediate medical help should be sought if a person has these symptoms.

Treatment: emergency medical treatment and intensive care in hospital will be required. This involves attempting to restore a normal heartbeat by means of electric shock and drug treatment. The drugs that may be used include digoxin, betablockers and calcium antagonists. Surgery and the fitting of a pacemaker is sometimes (but rarely) required. Underlying heart disease, responsible for the atrial fibrillation, is also treated, although this is rarely sufficient to restore the normal heartbeat on its own. An exception is if the cause is hyperthyroidism. Later, the patient may be prescribed blood-thinning drugs such as warfarin.

Causes and risk factors: in atrial fibrillation, the output of the heart is maintained by the contraction of the ventricles (the lower, larger chambers) alone. It can arise spontaneously in persons with no apparent heart disease, but often an underlying disorder is present. These diseases include coronary artery disease, rheumatic heart disease, atherosclerosis, high blood pressure (hypertension) and overactive thyroid gland (hyperthyroidism). There is a risk of CORONARY THROMBOSIS because of the formation of blood clots in the heart.

bends, the *see* CAISSON DISEASE

bleeding *see* HAEMORRHAGE

blood clot *see* EMBOLISM, THROMBOSIS

blood poisoning or **septicaemia**
Description: a serious and potentially life-threatening condition characterised by the presence of pathogenic microorganisms (especially bacteria) in the blood.

Persons most commonly affected: all age groups and both sexes.

Organ or part of body involved: blood circulation and all body systems.

Symptoms and indications: a temperature that rises rapidly to a high level along with shivering chills, flushing, copious sweating, pains and aches, and a fall in blood pressure. The person feels generally unwell and requires prompt medical attention as there is a risk of shock and death. This is especially the case in a vulnerable person who has an existing illness.

Treatment: involves admittance to hospital and antibiotic therapy. Antibiotics may be required in large amounts until the condition is brought under control. If blood poisoning has arisen as a result of infection in some other organ or part of the body (e.g. the gall bladder), surgery may be necessary to treat this.

Causes and risk factors: blood poisoning may result from infection in a wound or operation site or a tooth abscess. Also as a result of an infection in the gall bladder, appendix, burns or abscesses. Elderly persons and babies are more at risk, and people with lessened immunity, e.g. those suffering from cancer. Preventative measures include seeking prompt medical attention for infections, wounds and injuries, and having regular dental checkups and treatment.

bone fracture *see also* page 45
Description: any break in a bone, which may be complete or incomplete. There are many different forms of fracture, and these are listed below:

- Simple fracture (or closed fracture). In this type, the skin remains more or less intact.
- Compound fracture (or open fracture). An open wound connects the bone with the surface. This type of fracture is more serious as it provides a greater risk of infection and more blood loss.
- Pathological fracture. A fracture in a diseased bone, which often occurs in people, especially women, with osteoporosis.
- Stress fracture. Occurs in a bone that suffers re-current, persistent stress e.g. the march fracture sometimes seen in the second toe of soldiers after long marches.
- Greenstick fracture. This occurs only in young children, whose bones are still soft and tend to bend. The fracture occurs on the opposite side to the causal force.
- Complicated fracture. This involves damage to surrounding soft tissue including nerves and blood vessels.

- Depressed fracture. This refers only to the skull when a piece of bone is forced inwards and may damage the brain.
- Comminuted fracture. A serious injury to a bone in which more than one break occurs, accompanied by splintering and damage to the surrounding tissues. It usually results from a crushing force with damage to nerves, muscles and blood vessels, and the bone is difficult to set.

Persons most commonly affected: all age groups and both sexes.

Organ or part of body involved: bones.

Symptoms and indications: symptoms include pain, bruising, swelling and bleeding. Also, if nerves are damaged there may be numbness or even paralysis below the level of the injury. If a limb is fractured there is severe pain on movement and an inability to perform normal activities, and the affected limb may appear deformed or rotated. Occasionally there may be a loss of pulse below the fracture site, particularly in the region of the hands and wrists or feet and ankles. Immediate and often emergency medical attention is needed if a person has a fracture or suspected fracture.

Treatment: involves admittance to hospital where X-rays (radiography) are taken to determine the nature and extent of the injury. Surgery is often necessary to repair or set a fracture and the bone or body part is usually immobilised, generally by means of a plaster cast and splints. Sometimes traction is needed, which involves the use of weights and pulleys to apply a pulling force. This ensures that the bone is kept in correct alignment while healing takes place. Once recovery is well under way, physiotherapy is often needed to restore movement.

Causes and risk factors: with more serious and complex fractures particularly, healing may take a long time or be only partial. Also, there may be shock and death because of HAEMORRHAGE if the injury is severe. There may be damage or obstruction of arteries causing problems in blood circulation or embolism. Fractures are caused by trauma to the bone through accident or injury or repeated stress.

botulism

Description: the most dangerous type of food poisoning, caused by the anaerobic (living without oxygen) bacterium *Clostridium botulinum*.

Persons most commonly affected: all age groups and both sexes but less common in children.

Organ or part of body involved: central nervous system and muscles.

Symptoms and indications: symptoms may appear within a few hours of eating food contaminated by the bacteria and/or their toxin. These include a dry mouth, blurred vision, constipation, retention of urine and dilation of the pupils of the eye. This leads on to muscle weakness and paralysis and may be fatal. Death results from paralysis of the muscles involved in respiration. If botulism is suspected, emergency medical help should be summoned immediately.

Treatment: requires admittance to hospital for intensive care nursing, which may involve the need for a ventilator. Also, drugs that counter the effects of the bacterial toxin are given.

Causes and risk factors: the bacteria that cause botulism grow in tinned foods that have not been properly preserved, especially canned raw meats, fish, vegetables or fruit. Very rarely, infection may occur via an open wound or cut. During its growth the bacteria produce a toxin, one component of which attacks the nervous system and produces the symptoms. The toxin is destroyed by heat so it is a problem only in foods that have not been thoroughly cooked. The toxin has a very small lethal dose, hence it is a wise precaution never to taste suspect food but to discard it immediately.

brain compression

Description: pressure or squeezing of the brain within the limited space of the skull, due to some form of trauma or injury.

Persons most commonly affected: all age groups and both sexes.

Organ or part of body involved: brain.

Symptoms and indications: symptoms include drowsiness, breathing difficulties, weak pulse, paralysis in one side of the body and unconsciousness. Emergency medical treatment is needed if a person shows signs of brain compression.

Treatment: involves admittance to hospital and a surgical operation (trepanning or trephining of the skull – removal of an area of bone) so that the cause of the compression can be dealt with.

Causes and risk factors: there are various reasons why compression of the brain occurs. These include injury and rupture of a blood vessel producing a clot, tumour and a collection of pus or blood from an infection. As with brain abscess, preventative measures include seeking prompt medical attention for any injury, wound or trauma involving the head and skull.

burns and scalds *see also* page 24

Description: burns are damage to the skin and underlying tissues caused by dry heat, and scalds are similar injuries caused by wet heat. Formerly, burns were categorised by degrees (first, second and third) but are now usually described either as superficial, where sufficient tissue remains to ensure that the skin regrows, or deep, where grafting will be necessary.

Persons most commonly affected: all age groups and both sexes.

Organ or part of body involved: skin and underlying tissues.

Symptoms and indications: symptoms depend on the severity of the burn or scald. If it is relatively minor, there is pain and reddening of the skin, which may later blister or become white and peel off. In more severe burns there are raw wounds from which the skin peels off with a loss of fluid from the injury. Severe wounds of this nature can lead to shock and death, due to fluid loss at the burn site, and infection. All but the most minor burns should be seen by a doctor. In the case of extensive or severe burns and scalds, emergency medical help should be called.

Treatment: depends on the nature and severity of the burn or scald. Minor injuries can be effectively treated by running the affected part under cold water and then covering it with a dressing if needed. Slightly more severe burns should be treated by a doctor and require careful dressing and the use of antiseptics and antibiotics to combat likely infection. Serious and extensive burns are life-threatening and require emergency treatment, the most important part of which is transfusions to counter the fluid loss and maintain the circulation. The person is usually given strong pain relief, such as morphine, and antiseptics and antibiotics are needed to combat infection. Recovery is usually slow, and once the critical period is past, the person is likely to require skin grafting. The greater the extent of the burns and their depth, the poorer the chances of survival, and children and elderly persons are especially vulnerable. Chemical burns require special treatment to counteract the effects of the chemical involved.

Causes and risk factors: burns are caused by dry heat such as fire, sunburn, hot oil or fat in cooking, and also electrical currents and chemicals. Scalds are caused by very hot or boiling water and steam. Small children and the elderly are especially vulnerable to the risk of accidental burns in the home. Hence, the aim should be one of prevention and vigilance to eliminate areas of risk e.g. use of fire-guards, cooker guards, safety kettles kept out of reach, fire-retardant clothing (especially pyjamas and nightdresses), installing smoke alarms and general awareness of fire danger.

bursitis

Description: inflammation of a bursa (a fluid-filled hollow surrounding and protecting a joint) e.g. housemaid's knee.

Persons most commonly affected: adults of all age groups and both sexes.

Organ or part of body involved: bursae of joints, especially the knees, elbows, shoulders, wrists, ankles.

Symptoms and indications: pain, especially on moving the affected part, resulting in restriction of normal activity. Also, there may be some swelling and heat. A person with symptoms of bursitis should seek medical advice.

Treatment: the most important aspect of treatment is to rest the affected part and avoid the activity that caused the condition, if this is known. Also, an injection of a corticosteroid preparation into the bursa may be needed to reduce inflammation.

Causes and risk factors: the cause may be obvious, as in the case of housemaid's knee, which is caused by excessive kneeling. Or there may be other repetitive activities that have put the joint under too much strain. However, sometimes the cause of the condition is less easy to discern. Occasionally, there may be infection in the bursa, which is then treated in the same way as an abscess.

Caisson disease or **compressed air illness** or **'the bends'**

Description: a condition suffered by persons operating in high pressure in diving bells or divers at depth underwater if they surface too rapidly. Also, those who fly fast, high-performance aircraft.

Persons most commonly affected: adults who are divers or who work in the conditions outlined above e.g. in the oil industry, military aircraft.

Organ or part of body involved: blood and tissues throughout the body.

Symptoms and indications: pains in the joints (the bends), headache and dizziness (decompression sickness), chest pain, breathing difficulties, unconsciousness. Paralysis and death may occur if the person does not receive emergency medical attention.

Treatment: involves admittance to hospital, or a facility with a decompression chamber, until the person has recovered and been slowly readjusted to normal surface pressures.

Causes and risk factors: the cause of this condition is the formation of nitrogen bubbles in the blood, which then accumulate in different parts of the body. The nitrogen bubbles hinder the normal circulation of the blood in supplying the tissues with nutrients and oxygen. Treatment in a decompression chamber forces the nitrogen bubbles to redissolve into the blood. There is a risk of damage to the bones, lungs, brain and heart because of the interruption of the blood circulation, particularly if the person is severely or repeatedly affected. Those working in the occupations listed above, or who take up scuba diving, should receive adequate training and have access to proper medical facilities. The condition can be avoided by returning slowly from high to lower pressure, spending adequate time at each level.

carbon monoxide poisoning

Description: carbon monoxide is an odourless and colourless gas that is highly dangerous when inhaled, leading to carbon monoxide poisoning.

Persons most commonly affected: all age groups and both sexes.

Organ or part of body involved: blood, all tissues and brain.

Symptoms and indications: the symptoms of poisoning include giddiness, flushing of the skin (due to carboxyhaemoglobin in the blood, which is bright red), nausea, headache, raised respiratory and pulse rate and eventual collapse, coma, respiratory failure and death. Carbon monoxide poisoning is an emergency and the person requires immediate medical help.

Treatment: the most important treatment is to immediately remove the person into fresh air and start artificial respiration if needed. Other emergency medical treatment may be needed in the form of giving of oxygen and assisted ventilation.

Causes and risk factors: in the blood, carbon monoxide has a much greater affinity for oxygen (300 times higher) than haemoglobin and converts haemoglobin into carboxyhaemoglobin. (Haemoglobin is the red pigment present in the blood that picks up oxygen in the lungs and carries it in the circulation to all the tissues and organs of the body.) The tissues and organs of the body are quickly deprived of oxygen because there is no free haemoglobin left to pick it up in the lungs. Permanent damage is eventually caused to the ganglia at the base of the brain. Carbon monoxide is present in coal gas fumes and the emissions of vehicle exhausts. Domestic cases of accidental poisoning usually occur due to inadequate ventilation and ineffective maintenance of boilers and heating systems.

cardiac arrest *see also* pages 69–82

Description: the failure and stopping of the pumping action of the heart.

Persons most commonly affected: adults of all age groups and both sexes but particularly middle-aged and elderly persons. Less common in premenopausal women than in men but same incidence in women after menopause as in men.

Organ or part of body involved: heart.

Symptoms and indications: loss of consciousness, breathing and pulse stops, skin is pale and tinged with blue, pupils become dilated. Cardiac arrest or heart attack is a medical emergency and a person requires immediate aid.

Treatment: involves attempting to restart the heart by external cardiac massage (direct depressions of the breastbone *see* p.76) along with artificial respiration (mouth-to-mouth resuscitation *see* p.74). In hospital, defibrillation (electric shock) and direct cardiac massage (the chest wall is opened to allow massage of the heart) may be attempted as a last resort.

Causes and risk factors: causes include various forms of heart disease e.g. CORONARY THROMBOSIS, heartbeat irregularities, serious electrolyte (salts)/ fluid imbalance and shock due to severe injury and HAEMORRHAGE. Also, electrocution, ANAPHYLACTIC

SHOCK, lack of oxygen and respiratory arrest. Stress is believed to be a contributory factor, especially in people with existing heart disease or who are otherwise susceptible.

cauliflower ear

Description: a thickening of the external part of the ear that can lead to permanent deformity, caused by repeated injury suffered in sport.

Persons most commonly affected: men, especially those who are, or have been, boxers.

Organ or part of body involved: ear.

Symptoms and indications: a collection of blood (haematoma) following a blow or blows on the ear while playing sport. A person with the injury requires medical treatment as soon as possible to prevent permanent deformity.

Treatment: usually requires admittance to hospital where the blood is released to reduce the swelling. A firm bandage, which applies pressure to keep the swelling down, is then used. It is advisable to protect the ears and head during sports activities.

Causes and risk factors: thickening and deformity of the ears is a common injury among boxers.

compressed air illness *see* CAISSON DISEASE

concussion

Description: a loss of consciousness due to a blow to the head, causing bruising of the brain.

Persons most commonly affected: all age groups and both sexes.

Organ or part of body involved: brain.

Symptoms and indications: the symptoms vary in severity and reflect, to some extent, the force of the blow. There may be confusion, headache and dizziness in a case of mild concussion, or the person may fall into unconsciousness and remain in that state for seconds, hours or even weeks. It may be possible to rouse the person to some extent, but he or she is extremely irritable and does not answer questions correctly and soon becomes unconscious again. When the person comes round from the state of unconsciousness he or she usually suffers from a severe headache and irritability and these symptoms can last for some time. A person suffering from concussion usually needs to be admitted to hospital and a doctor should be called.

Treatment: depending upon the severity of the concussion, the patient requires admittance to hospital for rest and observation. There is a danger of bleeding caused by the blow on the head, which could result in serious, life-threatening damage to the brain. When the unconsciousness persists for some time the person requires careful monitoring, nursing and observation. Once the person has regained consciousness, even in mild cases of concussion, rest is needed until the headache subsides.

Causes and risk factors: the cause of concussion is a sudden knock to the head causing a compression wave that momentarily interrupts the blood supply to the brain. As indicated above, there is a risk of bleeding and further brain damage. The person normally makes a good and complete recovery but there may be memory loss, irritability and a tendency to headaches, lasting for several months. Also, there may be a risk or tendency in some people to epilepsy.

convulsions or **fits** *see also* pages 37–40
Description: involuntary and rapidly alternating muscular contractions and relaxations throwing the body and limbs into contortions. Convulsions are themselves a symptom triggered by some underlying cause.

Persons most commonly affected: babies from about the age of six months and young children up to four years. Both sexes may be affected. Convulsions can also affect adults of both sexes.

Organ or part of body involved: brain and central nervous system; muscles.

Symptoms and indications: in young children, convulsions usually accompany a fever. Hence, the child is often already unwell and feverish. During the convulsion itself, there is uncontrolled twitching and jerking of the limbs, body, head and face, and unconsciousness. The person may lose control of bladder and bowel function and be irritable on regaining consciousness. Following the convulsion, the person usually sleeps for several hours. The convulsion normally only lasts for a few minutes. A person who has had a convulsion should be seen by a doctor.

Treatment: depends upon the underlying cause of the convulsion. If triggered by fever, as is often the case in young children, measures to reduce the temperature and treat any infection are usually required. If the underlying cause is EPILEPSY, as is commonly the case in adults, then this requires appropriate treatment. If the convulsions continue, an injection of barbiturates or other sedative drug may be required.

Causes and risk factors: as indicated above, the commonest cause of convulsions in young children is fever. However, breath-holding, which is quite common in infants and very young children, is another cause. Also, breathing difficulties, which may occur, for example, during a bout of whooping cough, may trigger a convulsion. More serious causes include inflammation and diseases of the brain such as MENINGITIS and ENCEPHALITIS, and HEAD INJURY. In adults, the commonest cause is epilepsy. Convulsions are alarming to observe but unless caused by a serious disease or infection, in themselves they are rarely life-threatening.

corneal foreign bodies

Description: a foreign body lodging on the cornea or outer surface of the eye.

Persons most commonly affected: all ages and both sexes.

Organ or part of body involved: cornea.

Symptoms and indications: intense irritation and watering of the eye and photophobia (profound sensitivity to light).

Treatment: removal of foreign body and application of antibiotic drops or ointment. An eye patch may be worn until any damage has healed (usually about 24 hours).

Causes and risk factors: usually dust or material thrown up by mechanical tools. Can be avoided by wearing suitable eye protection when at risk e.g. when riding a motor cycle or when using power tools. If foreign bodies are not removed quickly from the eye, serious damage may be caused to the sight.

coronary thrombosis or **heart attack** or **myocardial infarction** *see also* pages 69–82

Description: a sudden blockage of one of the coronary arteries by a blood clot or thrombus that interrupts the blood supply to the heart. This causes death of myocardial (heart muscle or myocardium) cells due to interruption of the blood supply.

Persons most commonly affected: men, especially aged over 40, but also occurs in women.

Organ or part of body involved: arteries and heart.

Symptoms and indications: severe and agonising chest pain that may spread to involve the left arm, upper back, neck and jaw. Breathlessness and a crushing feeling on the chest, vomiting and nausea. A rise in temperature and pale and clammy skin, rapid pulse and collapse. A person suffering a coronary thrombosis requires urgent medical help and the emergency services should be called. If the person stops breathing and the heart stops, mouth-to-mouth resuscitation and external cardiac massage must be given until help arrives. Provided that a person receives prompt medical help, and survives the critical hours following a first heart attack, a good recovery is possible and normal activities can be gradually resumed. However, a severe heart attack may be fatal and the outlook is less favourable if the onset of treatment is delayed.

Treatment: following admittance to hospital, consists of giving strong pain relief, such as injections of morphine, oxygen and thrombolytic drugs to break up blood clots. The person requires intensive nursing in a coronary care unit. Various other drugs designed to restore the function of the heart are likely to be required, including anti-arrhythmics, beta-adrenergic or calcium channel blockers, digitalis, nitroglycerin and other antianginal preparations.

Causes and risk factors: the cause is a final sudden blockage or occlusion of one of the coronary arteries that has previously become narrowed. This causes an interruption of the blood supply to part of the heart muscle, which dies, and this is known as myocardial infarction. The heart ceases to pump blood effectively, with the symptoms described above. The risk of heart attack increases with smoking, a poor diet high in fat and salt, obesity, high blood pressure (hypertension), stress, lack of exercise and raised levels of cholesterol in the blood.

croup *see also* pages 22–23

Description: a group of diseases characterised by infection, swelling and partial obstruction and inflammation of the entrance to the larynx, occurring in young children.

Persons most commonly affected: young children of both sexes up to the age of about six years.
Organ or part of body involved: larynx, windpipe (trachea) and bronchial tubes (leading to the lungs).
Symptoms and indications: harsh, strained breathing producing a characteristic crowing sound, accompanying a cough and fever. There may be pains in the chest or throat and the child is generally restless and unwell. Attacks usually occur at night. If the child is experiencing severe difficulties in breathing, emergency medical attention is required. Milder cases can be treated at home but a doctor should be consulted.
Treatment: mild cases can be relieved by taking the child into the bathroom and turning on the hot water taps to produce a steamy atmosphere. The condition can be relieved by inhalation of steam from a bowl or basin of hot water to which a soothing preparation, such as tincture of benzoin, can be added. Mild sedatives and/or painkillers may be prescribed by a doctor. The child should be encouraged to drink plenty of fluids. Rarely, the obstruction becomes dangerous and completely blocks the larynx. The outcome is rapidly fatal, unless the child has been admitted to hospital, where nasotracheal intubation or emergency tracheostomy to restore the airway can be carried out.

Causes and risk factors: diphtheria used to be the most common cause of croup but it now usually results from a viral infection of the respiratory tract (laryngotracheobronchitis), or less commonly, a bacterial infection. A child normally makes a good recovery from croup but attacks are likely to recur. The child should be discouraged from playing outside in cold, damp weather, as this may cause an attack in some cases.

delirium

Description: an acute mental disorder, in which there is disorientation, confusion and hallucination, with several causes.

Persons most commonly affected: all age groups and both sexes.

Organ or part of body involved: brain.

Symptoms and indications: incoherence, confusion, restlessness, fear, anxiety, often hallucinations or illusions and sometimes delusions. If the delirium is caused by alcoholism, it is called *delirium tremens*.

Treatment: usually by treating the cause. If this is fever, then sponging the patient with tepid water to reduce the temperature will help. Fluid intake and nutrition must be maintained, and if the cause is withdrawal from alcohol dependence, sedation may be required.

Causes and risk factors: a wide range of metabolic disorders, postpartum (after childbirth) or postoperative stress, ingestion of toxic substances, *see* p.85, (including alcohol), physical or mental stress or exhaustion may all cause delirium.

dislocation *see also* pages 53 and 65
Description: a bone wrenched out of place at a joint is said to be dislocated. If the dislocation is minor, it may be called subluxation.
Persons most commonly affected: all ages, both sexes.
Organ or part of body involved: any joint, but most commonly the jaw, shoulder, knee and spine. Some children are born with hip dislocation.
Symptoms and indications: the joint is very painful and swollen and may show bruising. There is usually difficulty in moving the joint.
Treatment: relocation of the joint by a doctor and then immobilisation of the joint for a few weeks. Occasionally, surgery may be required, but this is normally only if dislocations happen repeatedly.
Causes and risk factors: dislocation is usually accidental. It may sometimes be caused by a shallow or poorly formed joint surface (usually congenital) or arthritis.

drowning *see also* pages 34–36, 71–82

Description: the immediate aftereffects of prolonged submersion in water.

Persons most commonly affected: all ages and both sexes.

Organ or part of body involved: lungs, blood and heart.

Symptoms and indications: there is a lack of spontaneous breathing. The patient has a blue colour and has no pulse.

Treatment: the patient must be removed from the water. If there are any foreign bodies in the mouth, such as weed, mud or false teeth, they must be removed. A check must be made to determine whether the patient is breathing, and whether he or she has a pulse or not. Artificial respiration and external cardiac massage (cardiopulmonary resuscitation or CPR) must be started at once if required *(see* pages 71–82), and help sent for. The CPR should be kept up until either the patient recovers enough to breathe unaided, in which case they should be put in the recovery position, or until the emergency services arrive to take over.

Causes and risk factors: water entering the lungs. In 15 per cent of cases, submersion in water causes a spasm of the larynx. To avoid drowning accidents, learn to swim. Do not swim after drinking alcohol, or too soon after eating. Do not swim in deep water to cool down on a hot summer day, as the water may be very cold, resulting in a sudden and disabling cramp. Do not dive or jump into unknown water; there may be underwater obstructions like weed or rocks, or in a swimming pool, underwater hazards. Do not leave small children alone in the bath, or in gardens with ornamental pools, as a child can drown in just a few inches of water. When taking part in water sports, like boating or water-skiing, wear a life jacket.

drug poisoning/overdose *see also* page 85
Description: caused by accidental overdose or by the misuse of a mood-changing substance for pleasure. Drugs can be inhaled, swallowed or injected into the body. Some of the most common substances used are nicotine, alcohol (*see* ALCOHOL POISONING), amphetamines, barbiturates, cocaine, opium alkaloids, glues and solvents, cannabis and psychedelic drugs.
Persons most commonly affected: all ages and both sexes.
Organ or part of body involved: central nervous system, blood, liver and kidneys.
Symptoms and indications: these depend on the substance and the quantity taken, but most of them

give altered behaviour. There may be increased sensitivity to sights and sounds. In drug overdose vomiting will not always occur immediately but his should be a symptom that you are on the alert for. The pupils of the eyes will be abnormally contracted or dilated.The use of heroin and cocaine makes the pupils of the eyes contract to pinpoints.

Treatment: if the person is conscious, ask them what they have taken. If the casualty is unconscious place them in the recovery position (*see* pages 83–84) and obtain medical help immediately. If you know what the casualty has taken tell the hospital and, if you can, give them a sample of vomit and any pill bottles and boxes that you may find nearby.

Causes and risk factors: drug misuse causes the risk of accidental injury while under the influence of the substance. Drug abusers risk serious infections if using non-sterile needles for injected drugs, such as hepatitis, BLOOD POISONING and HIV. There is a high risk of death caused by overdose, and body organs may suffer irreversible damage.

dysentery (amoebic and bacillary)

Description: an inflammation of the intestine, especially the colon, caused by bacteria (bacillary dysentery) or protozoa (amoebic dysentery).

Persons most commonly affected: all ages and both sexes.

Organ or part of body involved: digestive tract, but especially the colon.

Symptoms and indications: bacillary dysentery: severe diarrhoea, with the passage of blood and mucus. There may be nausea, cramp and fever, and the symptoms may last for about a week. Amoebic dysentery: symptoms may appear within a week of infection, or may take years to appear. The onset is very gradual, with weight loss, anaemia and indigestion, and eventually, passing of bloody stools.

Treatment: bacillary dysentery; bed rest, rehydration with plenty of water, and great care to ensure that any soiled clothing or bedding is either destroyed or thoroughly cleaned and disinfected. Amoebic dysentery; treatment with nitroimidazole drugs, followed by diloxamide furoate.

Causes and risk factors: bacterial dysentery is caused by infection from bacteria, amoebic by infection by protozoa. Both can be avoided by protecting food from flies, avoiding contaminated water and taking care to see that sanitation is good. Known carriers of either disease should not be allowed to handle food. Complications in bacillary dysentery only occur in severe cases, when the intestine may perforate and bleed. This may also happen with amoebic dysentery, where there is also a risk of abscesses forming in the liver, brain, bone or testes.

eclampsia of pregnancy

Description: convulsions (fits) arising in pregnancy.
Persons affected: females during pregnancy.
Organ or part of body affected: cardiovascular system (blood system).
Symptoms and indications: an early sign is raised blood pressure, with headaches and marked swelling of the ankles. (Slight swelling of the ankles is quite common in the advanced stages of pregnancy.) There may be an unexplained weight gain. The condition can be confirmed by the presence of protein in the urine. If untreated, convulsions will follow. The condition is usually discovered when the mother is in the early stages of the disease, when it is called PRE-ECLAMPSIA.
Treatment: bed rest is necessary, with careful monitoring of the foetus. If the condition is severe, an emergency Caesarian section may be required.
Causes and risk factors: these are unknown. It is more likely to happen in a first pregnancy, or where the mother is older. The mother may also be obese, have had previous hypertension or have diabetes mellitus. She may also be carrying twins,

or a Rhesus-incompatible baby. No hereditary link has been established but it is recommended that a pregnant woman inform her midwife or doctor of any history of the condition in her family.

ectopic pregnancy

Description: a pregnancy where the fertilised egg grows outside the uterus, usually in one of the Fallopian tubes joining the ovary to the uterus. As the egg grows, it stretches the tube and eventually ruptures it.

Persons affected: females during pregnancy.

Organ or part of body involved: usually Fallopian tubes.

Symptoms and indications: if a period is two to three weeks overdue, sudden severe pain in the abdomen. Sometimes, there is less severe pain and bleeding from the vagina. If no action is taken at this stage, there may finally be collapse from bleeding into the abdomen.

Treatment: immediate admission to hospital for surgery to remove the affected tube. If the blood loss has been large, a blood transfusion will be necessary.

Causes and risk factors: an ectopic pregnancy is more likely to happen if the Fallopian tube has suffered previous damage from infection. It is also more likely if there is a contraceptive coil in the uterus. As only one tube is affected by an ectopic pregnancy, it is still possible to conceive again.

embolism

Description: blocking of a small blood vessel, usually by a thromboembolism, but occasionally by fat after a bone fracture, or by air after an injection or a diving accident. It is usually in the lung (a pulmonary embolism), but may be elsewhere.

Persons most commonly affected: all age groups and both sexes.

Organ or part of the body involved: circulatory system.

Symptoms and indications: for a pulmonary embolism, these are shortness of breath, a sudden cough and chest pain that may be slight to very severe. Sometimes the lips turn blue (cyanosis), or there may be blood in the sputum. In severe cases, there may be symptoms of shock or unconsciousness.

Treatment: X-rays are taken to check the position of the embolism, and anticoagulants are given to prevent further clots. In severe cases, a patient may be admitted to hospital for oxygen and anticoagulant therapy, and sometimes surgery may be needed to remove the clot.

Causes and risk factors: it occurs most often after

surgery and other treatment involving long stays in bed. It can be partially prevented by moving about as soon as possible after surgery, childbirth or injury. For some operations that carry a higher risk, anticoagulants may be prescribed before treatment. People who have had previous emboli may take regular anticoagulants. Large embolisms can cause sudden death, medium embolisms usually heal, leaving no permanent disability and small embolisms are usually harmless and often heal without their presence being recognised.

encephalitis

Description: inflammation of the brain.

Persons most commonly affected: all age groups and both sexes.

Symptoms and indications: initial symptoms include fever, headache and neck stiffness, generalised aches and pains, fatigue, weakness and irritability. As the condition worsens, the affected person may become confused and disorientated and there may be CONVULSIONS, paralysis and eventually coma. Anyone with the symptoms of encephalitis requires emergency medical attention as it is a serious, life-threatening condition.

Treatment: Although there is no specific treatment for encephalitis the condition can be improved by

relieving the pressure around the brain (it is increased pressure caused by the inflammation that causes the symptoms). Admittance to hospital is necessary for intensive medical and nursing care.
Causes and risk factors: encephalitis is most commonly caused by a viral infection of the brain which can also lead to the inflammation of the meninges and the development of meningitis. It can also be a complication of a number of infectious diseases such as measles and chicken pox. Japanese encephalitis is caused by the bite of an infectious mosquito. There is a risk of permanent brain damage resulting from the condition.

epiglottitis

Description: a relatively rare inflammation and swelling of the epiglottis (the cartilage separating the back of the tongue and the entrance to the airway, which closes off the airway when swallowing).
Persons most commonly affected: both sexes, usually children aged one to six, but may occur in other age groups.
Organ or part of body involved: epiglottis.
Symptoms and indications: fever, noisy difficult breathing, cough, excessive saliva and rapid pulse developing quickly over a few hours.

Treatment: admission to hospital and antibiotic therapy. If obstruction to breathing is severe, the patient may be need to be intubated (have a tube inserted into the airway) or in very severe cases a tracheotomy (an incision into the trachea) may be necessary. Oxygen is usually given.

Causes and risk factors: it is caused by a bacterial infection, but it is rarely transferred between children.

epilepsy *see also* pages 37–40 and CONVULSIONS
Description: a neurological disorder characterised by the occurrence of convulsions or seizures and a loss of consciousness or momentary loss of awareness.

Persons most commonly affected: all age groups and both sexes. Usually, it starts in children between the ages of 2 and 14 and quite frequently below the age of 5.

Organ or part of body involved: brain.

Symptoms and indications: there are several forms of epilepsy and usually the symptoms arise suddenly. Occasionally, the person has a warning that an attack is about to occur. This is called *aura epileptica* and takes the form of odd or unpleasant sensations of sound, sight or smell, a change of mood, or pain or trembling in the muscles.

Grand mal seizure: this affects all age groups and involves a sudden loss of consciousness. The person falls to the ground, the muscles are stiff and he or she has a rapid pulse, poor pallor and dilated pupils. The body is then thrown into spasm by violent jerking of the muscles. The person may gnash the teeth, bite the tongue and froth at the mouth, and the eyes roll in the head. Breathing is noisy and the person may lose control of the bladder and bowel function. The attack usually lasts up to a few minutes and the body then relaxes. The person may regain consciousness to a certain extent but is usually very confused and soon falls into a deep sleep that may last for a few hours. On waking, the person may be restored to normal or feel tired, subdued and depressed.

Petit mal seizure: this often occurs in children and is characterised by a loss of awareness. The person suddenly stops the activity in which he or she is engaged and looks blank and is not aware of his or her surroundings. There may be some odd muscular movements or changes of expression. The attack lasts for a very short time and the person usually comes round and resumes previous activity, often being unaware of the episode.

Temporal lobe epilepsy: the affected person suddenly changes and behaves in an abnormal and inappropriate way, becoming angry or aggressive or agitated. Such behaviour is unusual and abnormal for that person.

Focal epilepsy: one part of the body is thrown into muscular spasm, although this may spread to involve the whole body, but there is no loss of consciousness.

A person who has an epileptic seizure requires immediate medical attention (*see* pages 37–37).

Treatment: is tailored to each individual's requirements and the person will require monitoring and periodic checkups. Various anticonvulsive drugs are used to control epilepsy, including phenytoin, primidone, methoin, clonazepam, sodium valproate and carbamazepine. The type and dose that is most effective varies between individuals. A person who suffers from epilepsy should not drink alcohol and may not be allowed to drive until two years have passed without an attack. Usually, seizures can be prevented and controlled and a person suffering from epilepsy can expect to lead a normal life. However, the condition generally cannot be cured except in those cases where surgery or other treatment can correct a brain disorder.

Causes and risk factors: there are a number of different causes, including brain injury, tumour or inflammation, and infection, disorders of metabolism such as hypoglycaemia, brain haemorrhage and birth trauma. Many people suffer a fit or CONVULSIONS at some stage in life, but most do not develop epilepsy.

fever

Description: a rise in body temperature above normal (37.4°C orally, 37.6°C rectally). Also called pyrexia.

Persons most commonly affected: may affect all ages and both sexes.

Organ or part of the body involved: any part of body may be involved.

Symptoms and indications: at the outset a fever is frequently marked by shivering that can become quite violent. In addition, in the early stages there is accompanying headache, sickness, thirst, diarrhoea or constipation, and possibly back pains. This is usually followed by an increase in pulse and breathing, hot dry skin, a marked thirst and loss of appetite and reduced urination. In severe cases where the body temperature continues to rise, there will be delirium. Loss of strength and some wasting of muscles may occur in prolonged cases.

Treatment: because a fever is a symptom of another condition or illness, it is vital that the underlying condition is treated. At the same time, some steps may be taken in an attempt to reduce the body temperature directly. The affected person may be sponged with tepid water or placed in a bath in which the water temperature is gradually lowered.

Certain antipyretic drugs, such as paracetamol and quinine, act on the controlling centres of the brain causing greater heat loss through the skin.

Causes and risk factors: fevers are caused primarily by viral or bacterial infections and may occur with any infection, however minor. Fever is the primary outcome of many diseases caused by a toxin in the system e.g. scarlet fever or typhoid, and the toxins are produced by bacteria in the body. Fever may also be associated with tumours, autoimmune diseases or shock.

The risk increases in cases of poor nutrition, in areas with poor sanitation, or where there is polluted water. Delirium occurs above a body temperature of 40.5°C. Excessive fever or hyperpyrexia occurs at 41.1°C and is regarded as dangerous while death usually results if the temperature remains above 41.7–42.2°C.

fits *see* CONVULSIONS, ECLAMPSIA OF PREGNANCY, EPILEPSY

food poisoning *see also* pages 85–86 and BOTULISM
Description: poisoning resulting from eating con-

taminated foods or ingesting poisonous chemicals, fungi or berries.

Persons most commonly affected: both sexes and all ages.

Organ or part of body involved: primarily the digestive system.

Symptoms and indications: in general, food poisoning results in nausea and vomiting, diarrhoea, abdominal pain and possibly headache and fever. The symptoms and the time of onset vary with the type of food poisoning, but will usually commence between one and twenty-four hours of intake.

Staphylococcal food poisoning from meat, milk or egg products generates symptoms abruptly within two to eight hours and the attack is usually short-lived (three to six hours) with complete recovery. Only susceptible individuals (young, chronically ill or the elderly) are likely to be at risk. *Clostridium perfringens* is associated with food poisoning from meat and meals that are reheated, and symptoms are produced within eight to twenty-four hours.

Numerous species of *Salmonella* cause food poisoning with symptoms following eight hours to three days after ingestion. Such infections are found in the meat and/or milk of domesticated cows, pigs and poultry and also in uncooked or lightly cooked hen's eggs.

Treatment: in the main, treatment is more preventative than curative, i.e. affected foods should be avoided and preparation and storage of foods should comply with good practice and appropriate regulations. Depending upon the severity of the attack, treatment may just involve bed rest, or, if there is severe vomiting, intravenous infusions of electrolytes may be required. Thereafter, the diet should be bland until recovery is assured.

Causes and risk factors: *Salmonella* (and also *Listeria*) are bacteria causing the symptoms. Although the animals mentioned above may be infected, they do not necessarily display symptoms, but products made from them create the poisoning. *Salmonella* are generally killed by heating to 60°C for about 15 minutes. Staphylococcal and clostridial food poisoning are caused by toxins released by the bacteria and in these cases, heating does not destroy either the toxin (staphylococcal) or the bacteria (clostridial). It is therefore essential that hygienic conditions prevail at all stages of food production.

Although the number of outbreaks of food poisoning has increased over recent years, it is not usually a fatal condition, but certain groups of people will be at greater risk, i.e. babies and the very young, pregnant women, the elderly and the chronically ill.

fracture *see* BONE FRACTURE

frostbite
Description: damage to tissue caused by exposure to freezing conditions.
Persons most commonly affected: no one particular group.
Organ or part of body involved: the extremities: toes, fingers, etc.
Symptoms and indications: the first symptoms of frostbite are when the affected area, be it toes, fingers or face, goes white and numb and all feelings of cold or pain disappear. As the severity of the condition worsens, there can be blisters on the frozen area, with a hardening and blackening of the skin. Swelling of the tissue produces tingling and sometimes severe pain. In very serious cases, the affected part becomes swollen and discoloured (blue/grey) and infection may set in.

Associated symptoms include shivering, slurred speech and possible loss of memory.
Treatment: shelter should be found immediately. The affected area should *not* be massaged, but warmed by putting in warm water, clothing or

similar, but not by placing near an open fire or by applying direct heat. A general warming of the body may be required, by means of hot drinks and insulation e.g. a sleeping bag. Any blisters should not be opened and the affected area should be cleaned carefully. It may be appropriate to give antibiotics to combat infection and analgesics to relieve pain. Anyone with a badly affected foot should not walk.

Causes and risk factors: frostbite results from the formation of ice crystals in the tissues causing tissue injury or tissue death in an extreme case. It is therefore essential that anyone who may be at risk is well clothed and equipped for the conditions and if frostbite does occur, can seek shelter and assistance quickly. A possible risk is that dead or infected tissue, be it finger, toe, nose or ear, may have to be amputated, but in mild cases (usually called frosting) full recovery is possible.

haemorrhage *see also* pages 13–20
Description: haemorrhage means bleeding – a flow of blood from a ruptured blood vessel, which may occur externally or internally. A haemorrhage is classified according to the type of vessels involved: arterial H – bright red blood spurts in pulses from an artery. Venous H – a darker coloured steady flow

from a vein. Capillary H – blood oozes from torn capillaries at the surface of a wound. In addition, a haemorrhage may be primary, i.e. it occurs at the moment of injury. Or, it is classed as reactionary when it occurs within 24 hours of an injury and results from a rise in blood pressure. Thirdly, a secondary haemorrhage occurs after a week or ten days as a result of infection (sepsis). Haemorrhage at specific sites within the body are designated by special names, e.g. haematuria (from the kidney or urinary tract), haemoptysis (from the lungs) and haematemesis (from the stomach).

Persons most commonly affected: all age groups and both sexes.

Organ or part of body involved: any blood vessel.

Symptoms and indications: the symptoms are, obviously, bleeding from the blood vessels involved but this may only be apparent if the haemorrhage is external. Internal haemorrhage may produce a range of symptoms depending upon the part of the body involved and the person is likely to be seriously ill. Haemorrhage from a major artery is the most serious kind, as large quantities of blood are quickly lost and death can occur within minutes from organ failure and shock. A person with a haemorrhage needs emergency medical treatment and admittance to hospital.

Treatment: is aimed at arresting the bleeding. For an external haemorrhage there are four approaches to stopping the bleeding (*see also* pages 14–17).

1 Direct pressure on the point of the bleeding.
2 Direct pressure on the artery or blood vessel.
3 Raising the wounded part (if a limb).
4 Application of substances (called styptics) to help the blood to clot or to constrict the blood vessels.

Hot water at a temperature between 46° and 49°C and, also, water that is ice cold, can be helpful in this respect.

For internal haemorrhage, it is important to keep the person lying down, as the heart then pumps the blood with less force and the blood pressure is lowered. Also, the patient should be kept calm and warm until emergency medical help arrives. Morphine is often given by injection.

A person with haemorrhage will require further treatment in hospital, which may include surgery and blood transfusions, depending upon the nature of the injury or other cause of the condition.

Causes and risk factors: the most obvious cause of haemorrhage is a wound or other injury. However, there are many others, including ulcers or drugs that may cause inflammation or bleeding in the digestive tract, haemorrhage after childbirth

and certain diseases or conditions, such as hae-
mophilia.

headache

Description: a pain felt within the head. Most people experience headaches at one time or another
and the causes and significance of these vary tre-
mendously. *See* MIGRAINE.

Persons most commonly affected: all age groups
and both sexes.

Organ or part of body involved: head.

Symptoms and indications: pain or ache in the head,
the site of which varies according to the cause of
the headache. A headache is often a symptom of
illness or disorder. In this case, it may well be accompanied by other symptoms, such as nausea and
vomiting. A person with a severe headache should
seek medical advice if the pain persists or if wor-
ried in any way.

Treatment: depends upon the underlying cause. If
the headache is a symptom of an underlying disease or disorder, then this must be identified and
treated. Other forms of headache can be relieved
using painkillers such as paracetamol.

Causes and risk factors: there are many causes of
headache and some are more serious than others.
Common causes are stress, tiredness, feverishness

accompanying an infection such as a cold, an excess of close work involving the eyes, dyspepsia (indigestion and digestive disorders), overexposure to hot sun (sunstroke or HEATSTROKE) and hunger. Other more serious causes include uraemia and kidney failure, high blood pressure, rheumatic diseases, glaucoma, brain disorders and infections such as MENINGITIS, ENCEPHALITIS, small inflammation of the brain, tumour and ANEURYSM. Also, a headache is a common symptom following brain injury or concussion. The arteries that supply it with blood, meninges (membranes) that cover it and the fibrous partitions within the brain are capable of transmitting the sensation of pain. It is thought that stretching and dilation, or other pressure on the arteries (called the intracranial arteries) may be the cause of headaches due to the disorders or diseases listed above.

head injury

Description: any injury to the head that may or may not be accompanied by a wound or fracture of the skull.

Persons most commonly affected: all age groups and both sexes.

Organ or part of body involved: head.

Symptoms and indications: the danger of a head

injury lies with possible damage to the brain itself. Hence, there may be bleeding and swelling if there is a wound, but also other symptoms that indicate that the brain has suffered trauma. These include drowsiness, nausea and vomiting, confusion and memory loss, blurring of vision, lapses into unconsciousness, headaches, effects on the pupils of the eyes and irritability (*see also* CONCUSSION). A person who has suffered a head injury should always be seen by a doctor and may require emergency treatment and admittance to hospital.

Treatment: the person requires admittance to hospital for observation, and may need further treatment, including surgery, depending upon the nature of the injury and development of symptoms.

Causes and risk factors: normally caused by an accident of some sort. It is important to wear proper protective headgear and helmets when taking part in various sporting activities, such as cycling, horse riding, etc.

heart attack *see* CORONARY THROMBOSIS.

heart block

Description: a condition in which there is a failure in the conduction of electrical impulses from the natural pacemaker (the sinoatrial node) through the heart, which can lead to a slowing of the pumping action. There are three types: in first-degree (partial or incomplete) heart block, there is a delay in conduction between the atria (the two thin-walled, upper chambers of the heart) but this does not cause slowing. In second-degree heart block, there is intermittent slowing because not all the electrical impulses are conducted between the atria and ventricles (the lower thick-walled, muscular main pumping chambers of the heart). In third-degree (or complete) heart block, there is no electrical conduction, the heartbeats are slow and the ventricles beat at their own inbuilt low rhythm.

Persons most commonly affected: men in middle and older age and postmenopausal women. However, can occur in people in younger age groups.

Organ or part of body involved: the electrical conduction system of the heart, which regulates the contraction of heart muscle.

Symptoms and indications: slow, irregular heartbeats, blackouts (Stokes Adams syndrome) and possible heart failure. A person with symptoms of heart block requires medical treatment.

Treatment: for second- and third-degree heart block, treatment involves admittance to hospital and the fitting of an artificial pacemaker that overrides and replaces the natural pacemaker of the heart. Although there can occasionally be a problem with electrical interference to the artificial pacemakers, the treatment is, on the whole, highly successful and abolishes all symptoms.

Causes and risk factors: heart block is more common in elderly people where degenerative changes have occurred. However, it is sometimes an inborn (congenital) disorder or may accompany other forms of heart disease, such as myocarditis (inflammation of the heart muscle), coronary thrombosis, cardiomyopathy and heart valve disease. As with many forms of heart disease, risks increase with smoking, a poor diet which is high in salt and cholesterol, stress and lack of fitness and exercise. Also, persons with high blood pressure (hypertension), diabetes mellitus, an imbalance of salts (electrolytes) within the body and previous heart disease are at a greater risk of developing heart block. The use of certain drugs such as quinidine, digitalis and beta-adrenergic blockers increase the risk of heart block.

heartburn

Description: a burning pain or discomfort felt in the region of the heart and often rising upwards to the throat.

Persons most commonly affected: adults of all ages and both sexes. Pregnant women.

Organ or part of body involved: stomach and oesophagus (gullet).

Symptoms and indications: unpleasant burning sensation in stomach, gullet and throat.

Treatment: the treatment is relieved by taking antacid tablets or alkaline substances such as sodium bicarbonate.

Causes and risk factors: the cause is usually regurgitation of the stomach contents, the burning being due to the acid in the gastric juice. Also, it may be caused by inflammation of the oesophagus (oesophagitis) or ulcers in the oesophagus. In order to prevent heartburn, it is advisable to avoid overeating or food and drink that might lead to an increased production of stomach acid. These foods include spicy curries, acid fruits, alcohol and coffee. The risk of developing heartburn increases with age, obesity, excess consumption of alcohol, poor diet and some drugs, such as aspirin and preparations taken for arthritis.

heat exhaustion *see also* pages 88–90

Description: exhaustion and collapse due to overheating of the body and loss of fluid following unaccustomed or prolonged exposure to excessive heat.

Persons most commonly affected: all age groups and both sexes but more common in elderly persons.

Organ or part of body involved: all body systems.

Symptoms and indications: in the mildest form, which is heat collapse, blood pressure and pulse rate fall and this is accompanied by fatigue, lightheadedness and, possibly, muscular cramps. The person urinates less frequently and is usually pale, but the skin may be moist and the temperature near to normal. A person showing these symptoms should receive treatment immediately and be seen by a doctor.

Treatment: involves rest in the shade away from the sun and taking extra fluids. Drinks of salt solution may be required, or this may need to be given intravenously. Recovery is normally good, occurring in about one or two days.

Causes and risk factors: the cause of heat exhaustion is unaccustomed or prolonged exposure to excessive heat. It is more common in hot climates and results from excessive sweating, leading to loss of fluids and salts and disturbance of the electrolyte balance in body fluids. It can be prevented by gradual acclimatisation to the heat, especially if hard physical work is to be carried out, and drinking lots of fluids. The risk increases with gastrointestinal disorders where there has been vomiting and diarrhoea, and if conditions are humid as well as hot. Any illness such as diabetes may make this condition more likely to occur and elderly people should be especially careful (*see also* HEATSTROKE).

heatstroke or **heat hyperpyrexia** *see also* page 89
Description: a severe condition that follows over-exposure of the body to excessive heat.
Persons most commonly affected: all age groups and both sexes with elderly persons most at risk.
Organ or part of body involved: all body systems.
Symptoms and indications: failure of sweating and all temperature regulation, headache, muscular cramps, hot, dry skin and high body temperature. The heartbeat rate is rapid, and there is a loss of consciousness, followed by coma and death, which can occur quite quickly. The person requires immediate emergency attention to save his or her life and admittance to hospital.
Treatment: the body is overheated and must be cooled immediately by sponging or immersion in cool water, and fanning. The body may be wrapped in wet sheets. Once the temperature has returned to just above normal (38.9°C), the person should be dried and wrapped in a dry blanket. When consciousness returns, drinks and salt solutions are

needed or may have to be given intravenously.
Convalescence may take some time and it may not
be possible for the person to continue former activities in the prevailing climate.

Causes and risk factors: the cause of the symptoms is loss of fluid and salt through excessive
sweating, leading to disruption of the salt/water
balance, lowered blood volume, metabolic disturbance and shock. Preventative measures include
taking enough time for acclimatisation to the heat
and increasing the amount of fluids drunk. People
who are required to carry out hard, physical work
need to drink salt solutions to compensate for the
loss that occurs in profuse sweating.

hernia

Description: the protrusion of a part or whole of an
organ from out of its normal position within the
body cavity. Most commonly, a hernia involves part
of the bowel. There are various types of hernia described according to their nature and origin.

- Congenital hernia – present at birth, a common
  one being an 'umbilical hernia', in which abdominal organs protrude into the umbilical cord.
- Acquired hernia – occurs after birth, a common
  example being an 'inguinal hernia' in which part
  of the bowel bulges through a weak part of the

abdominal wall (known as the inguinal canal).

- hiatus hernia – the stomach passes through the hiatus (a hole allowing passage of the oesophagus) from the abdomen into the chest cavity.
- Reducible hernia – one that is freely movable and can be returned by manipulation into its proper place.
- Irreducible hernia – one that cannot be returned by manipulation into its proper place.
- Incarcerated hernia – one that has become swollen and fixed in its position.
- Obstructed hernia – one involving the bowel. The contents of the hernia are unable to pass further down and are held up and obstructed.
- Strangulated hernia – the most dangerous type, in which the blood supply has been cut off due to the protrusion itself.

Persons most commonly affected: all age groups and both sexes.

Organ or part of body involved: any organ may be involved except the liver and pancreas. Usually, however, a hernia involves the bowel and digestive tract.

Symptoms and indications: a protruding lump that often can be returned to its normal position by manipulation. (However, not all hernias produce a lump that can be felt on the body's surface.) There may be slight discomfort or pain and a feeling of weakness. A strangulated hernia is a life-threatening condition causing severe pain, feverishness and vomiting, and eventually turning gangrenous. This requires immediate emergency surgery as there is a risk of peritonitis and death. A person with symptoms of a hernia should always seek medical advice.

Treatment: a reducible hernia may be treated by pushing back into place and support. Curative treatment is by means of surgery to return and retain the protrusion in its proper place (hernioplasty). It may be necessary for a person to go on a diet or have other treatment to reduce the size of a large hernia before surgery is performed. Treatment and recovery from all but a strangulated hernia is usually good and complete.

Causes and risk factors: the cause of a hernia is a weakness or injury in retaining muscles or connective tissue. There may be a congenital weakness, or stretching and tearing may occur along a line of weakness, such as a previous operation scar (incisional hernia). The risk of development of a hernia increases with age, pregnancy and obesity, and also inappropriate lifting and straining. In the latter case, the hernia may appear suddenly but usually its development is gradual.

hiatus hernia

Description: a hernia in which part of the stomach passes through the hiatus (a hole allowing the passage of the oesophagus through the diaphragm) from the abdomen into the chest cavity.

Persons most commonly affected: adults of both sexes over the age of 50 but can affect younger people.

Organ or part of body involved: oesophagus, diaphragm, stomach.

Symptoms and indications: the symptoms are usually felt after eating a meal and include heartburn, wind and discomfort. A person with symptoms of hiatus hernia should seek medical advice.

Treatment: includes the taking of antacid preparations to alleviate the symptoms of heartburn, eating small meals, avoidance of hot, spicy foods and, as with all hernias, avoidance of straining. Corrective surgery may be required to repair the hernia.

Causes and risk factors: there may be a congenital or inborn weakness in the diaphragm or this may be due to pressure or injury. The symptoms of heartburn are caused by backflow of gastric juice from the stomach into the oesophagus. The risk of the development of a hiatus hernia increases with age, obesity and inappropriate lifting or straining of the abdominal muscles.

hip fracture *see also* pages 46–47, 54–57

Description: the hip joint is a 'ball-and-socket' joint made up of the head of the femur (thigh bone), which rests inside a deep, cup-shaped cavity (the acetabulum) in the hip bone. The hip bone (or innominate bone) is itself made up of three fused bones, the pubis, ischium and ilium, which form part of the pelvis. A hip fracture involves a break of some sort in the femur.

Persons most commonly affected: all age groups and both sexes but especially older persons, particularly women with osteoporosis.

Organ or part of body involved: femur and other elements of the hip joint.

Symptoms and indications: severe pain, swelling and inability to walk following a fall or injury. A person suffering this injury requires immediate emergency medical treatment in hospital.

Treatment: is by means of surgery to repair the joint, securing the damaged portions by means of steel pins. Elderly patients may need a hip-replacement operation. Convalescence and recovery may take some time especially in older people.

Causes and risk factors: the cause is an accidental injury or, in the elderly, a fall. Care should be taken to avoid the possibility of falls and the diet should include adequate amounts of calcium. Women should consider hormone replacement therapy after the menopause to minimise the risk of osteoporosis. As with all injuries of this nature, there is a risk of poor healing, infection, and damage to nerves and blood vessels, especially if the fracture is severe or complicated. These are particularly dangerous in elderly people.

hyperventilation *see also* page 23
Description: breathing at an abnormally rapid rate when at rest, resulting in a fall in the concentration of carbon dioxide in the blood.
Persons most commonly affected: all age groups and both sexes.
Organ or part of body involved: respiratory system, central nervous system and whole body.
Symptoms and indications: hyperventilation is characterised by rapid, shallow breathing and the person may be agitated and then feel faint with tingling or numbing sensation in the hands, feet and face. If not checked, the person falls into unconsciousness. A person suffering from these symptoms should seek medical advice.
Treatment: hyperventilation often accompanies extreme anxiety. The affected person must be reassured and helped to calm down and breathe normally. Breathing into and out of a paper bag is help-

ful (the expired air contains more carbon dioxide).
Hyperventilation may also occur if the carbon dioxide level in the blood is abnormally high due to
impaired gas exchange in the lungs, as in pulmonary oedema and pneumonia, and subsides when
these conditions are treated and controlled.
Causes and risk factors: hyperventilation may occur as a result of extreme stress or anxiety or a sudden shock, as a symptom of a panic attack. The
person may need counselling to deal with stress if
the condition is a recurring problem.

hypothermia *see also* pages 87–88
Description: hypothermia describes the bodily state
when the core temperature falls below 35°C due to
prolonged exposure to cold.
Persons most commonly affected: all age groups
and both sexes but especially likely in elderly persons.
Organ or part of body involved: whole body – all
metabolism.
Symptoms and indications: early signs of hypothermia include shivering and the heart works harder
to increase the flow of blood around the body. The
person feels cold, the body temperature drops and
there is mental confusion and tiredness. Eventually, shivering ceases and, with increasing chilling,

the function of the body organs becomes disturbed and cardiac output falls. The tissues require less oxygen as their functions start to fail, but eventually the heart is unable to supply even this reduced demand. The symptoms are a further drop in body temperature and unconsciousness, leading to death. A person suffering from even mild hypothermia requires emergency medical treatment.

Treatment: consists of warming the person to restore body temperature to normal. If the core temperature has fallen very low (below 28°C) great care has to be exercised in moving the patient, who is susceptible to ventricular fibrillation. Warming is done by means of insulating blankets, warm water baths, heating pads, etc. The person may be given warm moist air or oxygen to breathe. However, peritoneal, gastric or bladder dialysis with warm saline solutions may be needed to save the life of an unconscious patient who is very severely chilled. The salt and water balance of the body is disrupted and requires careful monitoring and appropriate treatment along with ECG monitoring of the output of the heart. The person requires intensive care treatment and nursing until consciousness returns and the body temperature approaches a normal level.

Causes and risk factors: the cause of hypothermia

is prolonged exposure to severe cold. This is an obvious problem outdoors in winter especially if there is a cold wind. However, people may suffer from hypothermia when wet, even if the weather is not severely cold, or in accidents involving falling into the sea or other very cold water. Elderly persons can suffer hypothermia in their own homes when heating is inadequate. Preventative measures include the obvious ones of preparing for outdoor winter activities by wearing adequate protective clothing. Elderly people must keep their homes warm or live and sleep in one room that can be kept adequately heated. In some surgical operations (heart and brain surgery) a state of deliberate hypothermia may be induced while a particular procedure is carried out.

intestinal obstruction and intussusception
Description: an obstruction of some part of the intestine or bowel, preventing the passage of food material. Intussusception is an obstruction caused by one part of the bowel slipping inside another part beneath it, much as a telescope closes up.
Persons most commonly affected: all age groups and both sexes. Intussusception is more common in young children.

Organ or part of body involved: the small and large intestine or bowel.

Symptoms and indications: abdominal swelling and constipation, severe cramping pain that comes and goes, and characteristic vomiting. At first the vomit is normal but later it contains bile and is green, and later still resembles faeces (faecal vomiting). Symptoms of intussusception are similar, but a child passes a jelly-like, blood-stained mucus. A person with these symptoms requires immediate, prompt medical treatment as a delay may be dangerous or even fatal. Nothing should be taken by mouth.

Treatment: involves admittance to hospital and, usually, surgery to remove the cause of the obstruction, or barium enema (intussusception). Recovery is usually good and complete in the case of intussusception, provided that the child receives prompt and early attention. Surgery to correct intestinal obstruction is also normally successful, especially when diagnosis and treatment begins early. However, a cure depends upon the underlying cause of the condition.

Causes and risk factors: intestinal obstruction has a number of causes, including the presence of a tumour pressing upon the area either within the bowel or in a near organ, scar tissue from previous lesions, infections or operations (adhesions), a swallowed object, e.g. a fruit stone or internal body such as a hard mass of faeces and a twisted bowel. There is a risk of abscess, perforation and peritonitis, which can prove fatal, particularly if treatment is delayed.

meningitis

Description: inflammation of the meninges (membranes) of the brain (cerebral meningitis) or spinal cord (spinal meningitis) or the disease may affect both regions. Meningitis may affect the dura mater membrane, the outermost layer or meninx, in which case it is known as pachymeningitis. Or, it often results as a secondary infection due to the presence of disease elsewhere, as in the case of tuberculous and syphilitic meningitis. Meningitis that affects the other two membranes (the piaarachnoid membranes) is known as leptomeningitis, which is more common and may be either a primary or a secondary infection. Meningitis is also classified according to its causal organism (viral or bacterial).

Persons most commonly affected: all age groups and both sexes.

Organ or part of body involved: central nervous system.

Symptoms and indications: the symptoms include

a severe headache, sensitivity to light and sound, muscle rigidity, especially affecting the neck, Kernig's sign (an inability to straighten the legs at the knees when the thighs are at right angles to the body), vomiting, confusion and coma, leading to death. These are caused by inflammation of the meninges and by a rise in intracranial pressure. One of the features of meningitis is that there is a change in the constituents and appearance of the cerebrospinal fluid and the infective organism can usually be isolated from it and identified. One of the most feared aspects of (bacterial) meningitis is that the onset of symptoms can be very rapid and death can also follow swiftly. A person with symptoms of meningitis requires admittance to hospital for urgent medical treatment.

Treatment: depends upon the cause of the meningitis, which is established by analysis of the cerebrospinal fluid. If the cause is a virus, the disease is usually less severe but may still prove fatal in some cases. Mild cases may recover spontaneously with bed rest in a darkened room. Some cases require treatment by means of antiviral drugs, such as acyclovir, given intravenously. If the cause is a fungal or yeast infection, the drug amphotericin B is normally given intravenously. Various bacteria may cause meningitis, especially those responsible for tuberculosis, pneumonia and syphilis. Treatment is by means of intensive doses of appropriate antibiotics and sulphonamide drugs given intravenously. The person requires additional treatment to correct dehydration and electrolyte disturbances and to lower fever.

Causes and risk factors: three types of bacteria are responsible for most cases of bacterial meningitis. These are *Haemophilus influenzae* type b, *Neisseria meningitidis* (meningococcus) and *Streptococcus pneumoniae* (pneumococcus). Meningococcus occurs in the nose and throat of about 5% of the population, who are carriers of the organism but rarely become ill themselves. Meningococcal meningitis is the most common form of the disease in children aged one year or under. Pneumococcal meningitis is the most common type in adults. In general, the very young and the very old are most at risk from meningitis but modern treatments and drug therapy have improved the outlook for recovery considerably.

migraine

Description: a very severe, throbbing headache, usually on one side of the head, and often accompanied by other symptoms.

Persons most commonly affected: adolescents and

adults of both sexes but especially premenopausal women.

Organ or part of body involved: head, eyes, gastrointestinal tract.

Symptoms and indications: early symptoms of a migraine attack may be nausea and disturbance of vision in the form of seeing flickering bright lights (the aura of migraine). A severe, throbbing pain develops, often sited over one eye, nausea continues and there may be vomiting. The person is sensitive to light and sound, which make the condition worse.

Treatment: consists of rest in bed in a darkened, quiet room until the symptoms subside (up to 24 hours), and taking pain-relieving drugs. Other drugs that may be prescribed are ergotamine tartrate and metoclopramide. An affected person may have to experiment to find which pain-relieving drugs are the most helpful. Usually, they are most effective if taken during the period when an attack is felt to be coming on.

Causes and risk factors: the cause is unknown but is thought to involve constriction followed by dilation of blood vessels in the brain and an outpouring of fluid into surrounding tissues. Migraine is a common condition and seems to be triggered by any one or several of a number of factors. These include anxiety, fatigue, watching television or video screens, loud noises, flickering lights (e.g. strobe lights) and some foods such as cheese and chocolate, and alcoholic drinks. There may be an inherited tendency for migraine and the most common time of onset is puberty. In women, attacks may no longer occur after the menopause.

peritonitis

Description: inflammation and, usually, infection of the peritoneum, a serous membrane (one lining a large cavity in the body) that lines the abdominal cavity. It may be acute or chronic (rare), localised or general. Acute, general peritonitis is the most dangerous form.

Persons most commonly affected: all age groups and both sexes.

Organ or part of body involved: peritoneum.

Symptoms and indications: pain in the abdomen, which usually rapidly becomes severe. There is shivering, chills and high fever, and the skin is hot. The abdomen swells and the muscles become rigid. Breathing is shallow and rapid, blood pressure falls and heartbeat rate rises. The symptoms may lead to shock and collapse and can prove rapidly fatal. A person with symptoms of peritonitis needs immediate emergency medical treatment in hospital.

Treatment: the underlying cause of the peritonitis must be identified and treated and this may involve surgery. Antibiotics are required to fight infection and fluids and nourishment are given intravenously. Recovery is likely, providing treatment begins at an early stage.

Causes and risk factors: the cause is usually bacterial infection, the organisms responsible gaining access either from an external wound (especially a deep stab wound) or from perforation of any of the digestive organs within the abdomen. Hence, inflammation of the stomach, gall bladder and bile duct (gallstones), bowels (obstruction or twisting), hernia (which may become strangulated), ulcers in the digestive tract that may rupture, APPENDICITIS, ECTOPIC PREGNANCY, pelvic inflammatory disease, pancreatitis, abscesses or cysts e.g. in the ovaries or Fallopian tubes, and infection following abdominal surgery all carry a potential risk of peritonitis. A form known as puerperal fever may occur in the first two days after childbirth, but is rarely serious, provided that the mother has access to hygienic conditions and good medical care. The chronic form of peritonitis is normally the result of tuberculosis. A variety of bacteria can cause peritonitis, particularly *E. coli*, which is normally present in the gut, staphylococci and streptococci.

Adhesions or scar tissue may form as a result of peritonitis, causing symptoms and problems later on.

placenta praevia

Description: attachment of the placenta in the bottom part of the uterus (womb) so that it may partly or completely cover the cervix. It occurs in about 1 in every 200 pregnancies.

Persons affected: pregnant women.

Organ or part of body involved: placenta (the temporary organ that develops during pregnancy and attaches the embryo to the uterus. It consists of both maternal and embryonic tissues and allows oxygen and nutrients to pass from the mother's blood to that of the developing baby. It secretes hormones that regulate the pregnancy and is expelled after the birth of the baby as the afterbirth.)

Symptoms and indications: there is a sudden onset of bleeding late in the pregnancy, which, although painless, may become severe. Bright red blood is passed. A pregnant woman with bleeding of this nature requires emergency admittance to hospital.

Treatment: placenta praevia resembles abruptio placenta and normally, an abdominal ultrasound scan is necessary to confirm the diagnosis. If the bleeding is not severe but only minor, and the pregnancy is not near to term, the patient is usually kept in bed for observation. If the bleeding is severe, the mother will require blood transfusions and the baby is delivered, usually by Caesarian section. Occasionally, vaginal delivery may be possible.

Causes and risk factors: the cause is not known but the risk increases in women who have had several pregnancies, have fibroids in the uterus or other abnormalities e.g. scarring that prevents normal attachment, and are in an older age group. The bleeding occurs because the placenta partially or completely detaches from the uterus, and may be triggered by changes as the pregnancy nears full term, such as dilation of the cervix, which occurs just before labour begins. There is a risk to the life of the mother due to the blood loss if admittance to hospital is delayed. The baby may not survive if very premature at the time of delivery.

pleurisy or **pleuritis** *see also* pages 21–23
Description: inflammation of the pleura, the serous membrane (one that lines a body cavity) that covers the lungs (visceral) and the inside of the chest wall (parietal). The membranes normally have a smooth surface that is moistened to allow them to slide over each other.

Persons most commonly affected: all age groups and both sexes.

Organ or part of body involved: pleura.

Symptoms and indications: generally, a chest pain that starts suddenly and varies in severity from relatively mild to intense. The pain is of a stabbing nature and is worse with movement, breathing, and coughing. Hence, breathing is shallow and rapid and, eventually, a characteristic sound called pleural frictional rub may develop, which can be heard with a stethoscope. The sound may be of a crackling, rasping or grating nature. Fluid may collect between the two layers, called pleural effusion, and this tends to deaden the pain but may decrease lung volume through pressure so that breathing is even more laboured. Sticky fibrous material may be discharged onto the surface of the pleura, which can cause adhesions, although this does not occur in all forms of pleurisy. A person with symptoms of pleurisy should seek medical advice.

Treatment: depends upon the underlying cause of the pleurisy, and is likely to require admittance to hospital. It involves the use of various drugs, including analgesics, antibiotics and bronchodilators. Strapping of the whole chest with elastic bandages and the use of heat may be needed to ease pain. Measures to ease the coughing up of bronchial secretions (such as the use of humidifiers) may be advised. In some cases, drawing off or aspiration of pleural effusion is required via a small incision in the chest wall. This relieves distressed breathing by enabling the lung(s) to expand properly once more.

Causes and risk factors: there are a variety of causes of pleurisy including injury, especially fracture of a rib, respiratory tract infections e.g. pneumonia, bronchitis and tuberculosis, other diseases including systemic lupus erythematosus (SLE), rheumatoid arthritis, cancer and asbestos-related disorders. There is a risk of PNEUMONIA, collapse of the lungs and scarring as a result of pleurisy.

pneumonia

Description: a severe inflammation and infection of the lungs caused by many different kinds of bacteria, viruses and fungi. Most cases are caused by bacteria. It results in the filling of the air sacs (alveoli) of the lungs with fluid and pus so that they become solid and air can no longer enter.

Persons most commonly affected: all age groups and both sexes.

Organ or part of body involved: lungs, bronchi, bronchioles (the major and minor air passages supplying the lungs).

Symptoms and indications: symptoms vary in intensity depending upon how much of the lung is affected. They include chills and shivering, high fever, sweating, breathlessness, chest pain, coughing and there may be cyanosis. (In cyanosis, there is a blue appearance of the skin due to insufficient oxygen within the blood and tissues.) A sputum is produced that is often rust-coloured or may be thicker and contain pus. Breathing is laboured, shallow and painful. The patient may become drowsy and confused if cyanosis occurs and convulsions can occur in children. A person with symptoms of pneumonia requires immediate medical attention.

Treatment: may require admittance to hospital for antibiotics, which may need to be given intravenously in the first instance. The patient may require oxygen and analgesics to relieve pain, and measures such as tepid sponging to reduce fever. Fluids may need to be given intravenously. Amantadine and acyclovir may be given for viral pneumonia. Recovery from pneumonia depends upon the severity of the illness, and whether it occurs in a person who was previously well, or as a complication of existing illness. The elderly and very young and those with previous illness are most at risk, and it remains a major cause of death.

Causes and risk factors: pneumonia is usually

caused by a bacterial infection and numerous different kinds may be responsible. Commonly, *Streptococcus pneumoniae*, *Staphylococcus aureus*, *Chlamydia pneumoniae* or *Mycoplasma pneumoniae* are the causal organisms. The elderly and very young, persons with a depressed immune system e.g. transplant patients and those who have been treated for cancer, Aids patients, those with alcoholism and people with respiratory disorders, such as obstructive airways disease (asthma), are most at risk from pneumonia. The infection is usually caught by inhalation of airborne deposits containing the bacteria.

pneumothorax

Description: air in the pleural cavity between the two layers of the pleura (the double serous membrane that covers the lungs and the inside of the chest wall), which exerts pressure and causes the lung to collapse.

Persons most commonly affected: all age groups and both sexes (depending upon the cause).

Organ or part of body involved: lungs and pleura.

Symptoms and indications: symptoms vary greatly depending upon the nature and extent of the pneumothorax and whether underlying lung disease is present. They include a sharp pain in the chest that comes on suddenly and may travel to the shoulder and abdomen, breathlessness and a dry, barking cough. If severe lung disease is present there may be collapse and shock with respiratory and circulatory failure. A person with symptoms of pneumothorax should seek medical advice.

Treatment: depends upon the nature and degree of severity of the pneumothorax. A patient with a simple, small pneumothorax and who has no existing lung disease requires no special treatment other than to rest until symptoms subside. The air is reabsorbed naturally and the affected part of the lung re-expands. If a larger area of lung is involved, this may take some time and the person requires monitoring to ensure that there is no leak of fluid (pleural effusion) or development of fibrous deposits. For a more severe or complicated pneumothorax, where there has been an injury or the person has existing lung disease, or is elderly and generally at greater risk, admittance to hospital is needed. The person may require a chest tube and various drugs including pain relief. In some emergency cases, the air may need to be drawn off rapidly by means of a needle or catheter into the chest wall, in order to save life. A person who has more than one pneumothorax on the same side may eventually require surgery.

Causes and risk factors: causes include a penetrating external wound or internal injury e.g. a lung punctured by a fractured rib. Also, rupture of one or more small air sacs inside the lung due to diseases such as emphysema, asthma, tuberculosis, cystic fibrosis, inflammation and infection e.g. abscess or fistula in the lung. A simple pneumothorax may occur for no apparent reason or be associated, in some people, with taking part in high-altitude flight or deep diving.

pre-eclampsia of pregnancy

Description: a complication of pregnancy arising after the 20th week and characterised by high blood pressure (hypertension), fluid retention (oedema) and the presence of a protein (albumin) in the urine.
Persons affected: pregnant women.
Organ or part of body involved: whole body.
Symptoms and indications: the symptoms of pre-eclampsia are a blood pressure of 140 over 90mm of mercury (or greater), or a rise in systolic blood pressure of 30mm or diastolic blood pressure of 15mm of mercury. Also, fluid retention causing swelling, especially of the hands and/or face and the presence of albumin in the urine. The symptom that is most likely to be noticed by the patient is the fluid retention and this, and any other symp-

toms, should immediately be reported to the doctor. Other symptoms may be detected during routine antenatal check-ups.

Treatment: in very mild cases of pre-eclampsia, the woman may be treated at home, requiring complete bed rest and careful monitoring until blood pressure falls and symptoms improve. If the woman's condition does not respond or in any other than very mild cases, admittance to hospital is necessary. The patient is usually given a salt solution intravenously and also magnesium sulphate. The aim is to stabilise the woman's condition, to lessen the risk of convulsions and bring about a fall in blood pressure, and then to deliver the child. Other drugs may additionally be needed. Once the patient's condition has improved, labour may be induced and the baby delivered normally, or a Caesarian section may be required.

Causes and risk factors: the cause is unknown but is more likely to occur in a first pregnancy and in women with a history of high blood pressure or blood vessel disorders. There is a danger of the development of eclampsia of pregnancy and also, abruptio placentae, both of which are potentially fatal conditions. With prompt treatment, the outlook for mother and child is usually good.

prolapsed intervertebral disc or **slipped disc**

Description: intervertebral discs are thick, fibrous cartilaginous discs that connect and lie between adjacent vertebrae of the backbone. They permit rotational and bending movements of the back and make up approximately 25% of the length of the backbone, acting as shock absorbers and providing cushioning for the brain and spinal cord. Each disc has an outer fibrous layer over a pulpy centre. A slipped or prolapsed disc is caused by the inner layer being pushed through the fibrous layer to impinge upon a neighbouring spinal nerve-causing pain.

Persons most commonly affected: adults of both sexes in middle or older age.

Organ or part of body involved: intervertebral disc, usually either between the last two lumbar vertebrae (lumbago) or the lowest lumbar vertebrae and the five fused sacral vertebrae that form the sacrum (sciatica).

Symptoms and indications: pain in the lower part of the back, which may come on and worsen gradually or, more usually, is sudden and occurs during an activity that involves bending or sudden twisting of the backbone. A person with symptoms of a slipped disc should seek medical advice.

Treatment: depends upon the severity of the condition but involves bed rest on a flat, firm surface, possibly with manipulation and physiotherapy at a later stage. Epidural anaesthesia (an injection of local anaesthetic into the spine) may be required to relieve pain. Occasionally, surgical removal of the disc may be carried out.

Causes and risk factors: a slipped disc is more likely to occur in middle or later adult life and may be related to degenerative changes that take place. However, the condition is not unknown in younger adults. It is sensible to take extra care when carrying out movements or activities that might stress the back.

pseudorubella *see* ROSEOLA INFANTUM

pulmonary embolism

Description: a condition in which the pulmonary artery (leading from the heart to the lung) or a branch of it, becomes blocked by a clot or embolus, which is usually of blood, and rarely a clump of fat cells. The clot usually originates as a phlebothrombosis of a deep vein in the leg or pelvis. The seriousness of the condition is related to the size of the clot. The clot moves through the circulation, ultimately lodging in a part of a pulmonary artery. Large pulmonary emboli can be fatal, while smaller ones may cause tissue death of parts of the lung, breathing difficulties and symptoms of pleurisy.

Persons most commonly affected: adults of both sexes but can affect people of all ages.

Organ or part of body involved: a pulmonary artery or one of its branches.

Symptoms and indications: there is a sudden and often severe pain in the chest, breathlessness and a cough that may result in the bringing up of blood. There is a rapid heartbeat rate and the person feels anxious and restless. The person may be feverish or faint and there may be shock and death if the clot is large. Often there are symptoms of pulmonary hypertension. A person with symptoms of pulmonary embolism requires immediate emergency medical attention.

Treatment: involves admittance to hospital. Anticoagulant drugs such as heparin may be prescribed in less severe cases, or streptokinase to dissolve the clot. In other cases, emergency surgery may be needed to remove the clot. Pulmonary embolism occasionally arises as a complication of surgery, injury, especially bone fractures, pregnancy and childbirth, due to the formation of a clot in a deep vein of the leg or pelvis. Preventative measures for hospital patients include the wearing of elastic stockings and encouraging leg exercises and walking as soon as possible after surgery, and also the use of drugs to thin the blood.

Causes and risk factors: The risk of phlebothrombosis and pulmonary embolism is greater in those who smoke or are overweight and in older women taking oral contraceptives. Also, it is more likely in those with existing heart and circulatory disorders, in elderly persons aged over 60 years, and in those with sickle cell anaemia and some other diseases (polycythaemia).

pulmonary oedema

Description: a gathering of fluid in the lungs arising for a variety of reasons, especially as a result of congestive heart failure or mitral stenosis. It produces severe and life-threatening symptoms.

Persons most commonly affected: adults of both sexes, especially those in middle or older age groups.

Organ or part of body involved: lungs and heart.

Symptoms and indications: great breathing difficulties with shallow, rapid breaths, cyanosis (a lack of oxygen in the blood), anxiety, restlessness, and a feeling of suffocation. Also, there may be sweating, a cough, dry at first but then producing a pink-stained frothy sputum, a weak or pounding pulse and characteristic crackling sounds from the lungs (called rales) that can be heard through a stethoscope. There may be a collection of fluid in the hands and feet, low blood pressure (hypotension), and veins may become engorged and prominent. A person with these symptoms requires emergency medical treatment.

Treatment: admittance to hospital is required for immediate treatment aimed at saving life. This involves the giving of oxygen, and various drugs may be required including narcotics (morphine sulphate), nitroglycerin, diuretics, e.g. frusemide or ethacrynic acid, digitalis and dopamine. The underlying condition responsible for the pulmonary oedema will require appropriate treatment. The outlook is more favourable if treatment begins promptly.

Causes and risk factors: the usual cause is failure of the left ventricle of the heart (one of the lower larger chambers) or mitral stenosis. Other causes include poisoning with some drugs, such as barbiturates or opiates, fluids and blood given intravenously, kidney failure, stroke, head injury, inhalation of toxic fumes and near-drowning.

pulmonary valve stenosis

Description: narrowing of the pulmonary valve,

which controls the outlet from the right ventricle (one of the large upper chambers of the heart) to the pulmonary artery leading to the lungs. This leads to obstruction and a reduction of normal heart function.

Persons most commonly affected: both sexes and all age groups. The congenital form is likely to become apparent at or shortly after birth.

Organ or part of body involved: heart.

Symptoms and indications: symptoms are those of angina, along with fainting and signs of congestive heart failure. These include breathlessness, fatigue, fluid retention and a cough which may produce a pink and frothy sputum. Part of the heart may become enlarged. A person with symptoms of pulmonary valve stenosis should seek medical advice.

Treatment: unless the symptoms are very mild, treatment usually involves admittance to hospital for surgery to clear the obstruction and widen the valve.

Causes and risk factors: the cause is usually congenital but rarely it arises as a result of rheumatic fever.

rabies

Description: a very severe and fatal disease affecting the central nervous system, which occurs in dogs, wolves, cats and many other mammals. Human beings are infected through the bite of a rabid animal, usually a dog. The UK is currently free of rabies but it occurs in many countries throughout the world.

Persons most commonly affected: all age groups and both sexes.

Organ or part of body involved: brain and central nervous system.

Symptoms and indications: symptoms may begin from ten days up to a year, following a bite from a rabid animal. Usually, however, they begin after four to eight weeks, starting with depression and irritability. Swallowing and breathing difficulties develop, and feverishness, and there are periods of great mental excitement, increased salivation and muscular spasms of the throat that are very painful. Eventually, even the sight of water causes severe muscular spasms, convulsions and paralysis, with death following in about four days. A person who is bitten by an animal that may be rabid should immediately thoroughly cleanse the wound with soap or detergent and antiseptic to remove all traces of saliva, being especially careful about deep punctures. The wound should be covered with a clean dressing and then medical advice should be sought.

The appropriate authorities should also be notified so that the animal can be caught and dealt with.

Treatment: is by means of injections of rabies vaccine, antiserum and immunoglobulin. A person who has previously received rabies vaccine as a preventative measure, and who receives a bite, requires further injections. The incubation period for rabies enables effective treatment to be given. However, if symptoms start, the outcome is normally fatal (in 80 per cent of cases), although some people survive with vigorous supportive treatment.

Causes and risk factors: the cause of rabies is a virus that is present in populations of wild and feral animals in many countries of the world. Rabid animals exhibit one of two forms of behaviour, known as 'mad' or 'furious' rabies and dumb rabies. In the former, the animal may exhibit wild, uncontrolled behaviour, running around and snapping and biting if it is a dog, or losing its normal fear of humans and behaving unusually, in the case of a wild creature. In the other form, which is a more advanced stage of the furious type, the animal is more or less paralysed and drags itself around but may bite if cornered. Preventative treatment with rabies vaccine is advisable for all those living, working or visiting countries where rabies is endemic and who are likely to be in contact with animals. If prompt medical care is available, rabies is uncommon in human beings but remains one of the most feared diseases.

retinal detachment or **detachment of the retina of the eye**

Description: a hole or tear in the retina, the layer that lines the interior of the eye and contains light-sensitive cells and nerve fibres. The retina consists of two layers and when the tear is produced, the inner one becomes separated from the outer one and retinal detachment occurs. This is caused by fluid (vitreous humour) leaking through the hole, forcing the inner layer to become detached from the outer layer.

Persons most commonly affected: all age groups and both sexes, especially males.

Organ or part of body involved: retina, usually of one eye only.

Symptoms and indications: symptoms include the appearance of floating spots (floaters) before the eye, blurring of vision, flashes of light and loss of sharpness in the centre of the image. The person may appear to see a veil or curtain in the affected eye. Any person with these symptoms requires immediate emergency medical treatment in order to preserve sight in the affected eye.

Treatment: consists of admittance to hospital for surgery to seal the hole or repair the separation of the retina by means of electric current, which produces heat (diathermy) or cold (cryotherapy) using liquid nitrogen or solid carbon dioxide. At an early stage, laser treatment may be the preferred method. Occasionally it may be necessary to alter the shape of the eye to bring about healing. The condition can usually be cured if treated at an early stage but a delay in treatment may result in permanent partial or complete loss of vision.

Causes and risk factors: the causes are eye injury or a complication of eye surgery (especially the removal of cataracts) and the risk increases in those with short-sightedness (myopia) and diabetes mellitus. Also, older persons are at greater risk, as are those with a history of this condition. Malignant tumours of the eye may also be a cause of retinal detachment.

roseola infantum or **pseudorubella** or **exanthem subitum**

Description: an acute fever and skin rash that is highly contagious and affects babies and young children.

Persons most commonly affected: babies and young children aged six months to three years.

Organ or part of body involved: central nervous system, skin.

Symptoms and indications: the child suddenly develops a high fever of 103° to 105°F or 39.5° to 40.5°C, for which there is no obvious cause. The fever usually lasts about three to five days and convulsions may occur. The child is irritable and unwell. The fever normally reaches a peak and then subsides and this coincides in some, but not all cases, with the development of a red rash, mainly on the chest and abdomen. This normally subsides quite soon and by this time the child is evidently feeling much better. A child who develops a high fever should always be seen by a doctor. The doctor should be summoned urgently if the child has a convulsion or shows signs of dehydration.

Treatment: consists of measures to reduce fever, including the use of medicines containing paracetamol that are designed for young children, tepid sponging and cooling fans. The child should be encouraged to drink plenty of fluids. In rare cases, admittance to hospital may be required. The child normally recovers well after a few days.

Causes and risk factors: the cause is now thought to be, in many cases, human herpes virus type 6 (HHV-6), although there may be others.

ruptured eardrum

Description: a hole that may develop in the eardrum because of infection or injury. It may also be called perforated eardrum.

Persons most commonly affected: all ages and both sexes.

Organ or part of body involved: ear.

Symptoms and indications: there may be sudden deafness following acute otitis media or injury. Sometimes, there may be sudden relief of the pain of otitis media. There may be a discharge from the ear, and sometimes sufferers complain of tinnitus.

Treatment: a doctor will usually clean the middle ear and prescribe a course of antibiotics. The ear should be protected while showering. In children, a ruptured eardrum usually heals within two weeks; in adults, this may take a little longer.

Causes and risk factors: It can be caused by severe or untreated otitis media. It may also be caused by sudden high pressure applied to the eardrum, either while diving, from a slap on the ear, or by a sudden very loud noise. It may be avoided by wearing ear protectors in a very noisy environment. Otitis media should always be treated and cleared up, and no-one should scuba-dive without training.

scalds *see* BURNS AND SCALDS

sciatica

Description: pain in the sciatic nerve, which is felt in the back of the thigh, leg and foot.

Persons most commonly affected: adults of both sexes aged under 60.

Organ or part of body involved: sciatic nerve, affecting leg and foot.

Symptoms and indications: the symptoms may develop rapidly, due to an awkward, strained or twisting movement, such as lifting a heavy object. Or, they may begin more gradually, due to an underlying condition causing pressure on the sciatic nerve. Symptoms include stiffness and pain in the back, leg and foot, which can be severe. A person with symptoms of sciatica should seek medical advice.

Treatment: may be in the form of bed rest and painkilling drugs until the symptoms improve. Persistent pain and weakness may require admittance to hospital for corrective surgery depending upon the underlying cause of the condition.

Causes and risk factors: the cause may be inadvertent stressing of the back, due to an awkward movement. However, the commonest cause of sciatica is a prolapsed intervertebral disc pressing on the nerve root, but it may also be due to ankylosing spondylitis or some other conditions e.g. spinal tumour.

septicaemia *see* BLOOD POISONING

shock *see also* page 100
Description: acute, circulatory failure due to blood pressure in the arteries falling so low that blood is no longer supplied to all parts of the body. Hence the normal functions of the body can no longer take place and there is a risk of death.
Persons most commonly affected: all age groups and both sexes.
Organ or part of body involved: blood circulatory system and heart.
Symptoms and indications: shock may develop as a result of injury or illness. The signs are a cold, clammy skin, pallor, cyanosis (blue-coloured skin due to a lack of oxygen in the blood), weak, rapid pulse, irregular breathing and dilated pupils. The person may feel anxious or suffer from confusion or lethargy and there is a lack of urination. Blood pressure falls to a low level and may not be detectable by normal methods. A person in shock requires immediate, emergency medical attention.
Treatment: depends upon the underlying cause of the shock. If due to bleeding or loss of fluid, this

must be halted and the person is likely to require blood transfusion and fluids given intravenously. If it is due to severe infection, large doses of antibiotics are likely to be needed. The person may be given drugs to raise blood pressure. General measures include keeping the person warm and calm and lying down with the legs raised. The patient should be accompanied at all times and emergency artificial respiration may be needed if breathing stops.

Causes and risk factors: there are numerous causes of shock, including a reduction in blood volume due to internal or external bleeding, and loss of fluid from burns or illnesses that cause dehydration and fluid/salt imbalance. Also, reduced heart activity as in coronary thrombosis, pulmonary embolism and heart rhythm disorders, blood poisoning and anaphylactic shock. Shock is a serious, life-threatening condition and the outcome depends upon the severity of the cause and response to treatment.

slipped disc *see* PROLAPSED INTERVERTEBRAL DISC

stroke or apoplexy
Description: the physical effects, involving some form of paralysis, that result from damage to the brain due to an interruption in its blood supply. The

effect in the brain is secondary and the cause lies in the heart or blood vessels and may be a thrombosis, embolus or haemorrhage. The severity of a stroke varies greatly from a temporary weakness in a limb, or tingling, to paralysis, coma and death.

Persons most commonly affected: elderly adults of both sexes although younger people may occasionally be affected.

Organ or part of body involved: brain.

Symptoms and indications: symptoms vary according to the nature and severity of damage to the brain and may be gradual or sudden in their onset. They include loss of control over movement, numbness or tingling on one side of the body, loss of speech, mental confusion and disturbance of vision, headache, loss of consciousness, with noisy breathing. The unconscious person may appear flushed and have a slow pulse rate, and the pupils of the eyes are unequally contracted. A person with symptoms of a stroke requires emergency medical treatment in hospital.

Treatment: is in the form of intensive nursing aimed at maintaining the person in as stable a state as possible. Some drugs might be given depending upon the nature of the stroke and the patient's condition. These include drugs to lower blood pressure, anticoagulants or heparin and nimodipine.

Physiotherapy and exercises of paralysed limbs, etc, are usually begun as soon as possible. A severe stroke often proves fatal. Patients who survive are likely to suffer physical and possibly mental disability and require a great deal of continuing help, support and encouragement.

Causes and risk factors: the cause of stroke is usually atherosclerosis, or hardening and narrowing of the arteries, which occurs with increasing age. This can result in a blockage of a small artery by a blood clot interrupting the blood flow to the brain (THROMBOSIS). Or, there may be an embolism in which a clot or plug is carried from the heart or an artery elsewhere, via the circulation to lodge in a vessel of the brain and cause blockage. Another cause of stroke is haemorrhage of a blood vessel within the brain, causing an escape of blood into the brain tissue. The blood vessels may already have become diseased and the leakage of blood may be due to rupture of an aneurysm. In a younger person who suffers a stroke, the cause is usually the rupture of an aneurysm (which has occurred due to some congenital weakness) leading to a subarachnoid haemorrhage.

subarachnoid haemorrhage

Description: bleeding into the subarachnoid space

of the brain. (The subarachnoid space occurs between two of the membranes or meninges that cover the brain, the arachnoid and pia-mater membranes. The space usually contains cerebrospinal fluid.)

Persons most commonly affected: adults of both sexes between the ages of 25 and 50 but can affect people in any age group.

Organ or part of body involved: brain.

Symptoms and indications: symptoms include a sudden, very severe headache, nausea and vomiting, dizziness, fainting and coma. Sometimes the person may suffer fits and heartbeat and breathing rates are erratic. Within 24 hours, the person develops a stiff neck and certain other muscle and reflex responses (called Kernig's sign and Babinski's sign). During the first few days after the haemorrhage, the person continues to suffer from headache and confusion and has an elevated temperature. There may be paralysis on one side of the body (hemiplegia). A person with symptoms of a subarachnoid haemorrhage requires emergency medical treatment in hospital.

Treatment: following admittance to hospital, diagnostic tests and scans are carried out to determine the nature of the haemorrhage. Treatment is usually by means of surgery to stop the bleeding e.g. by clipping an aneurysm. The outlook is best in patients who are well enough to undergo surgery within the first 72 hours. A majority of patients survive a first subarachnoid haemorrhage but there is a risk of a second one occurring, especially within the first few weeks. Surgery reduces the risk of subsequent haemorrhage. Patients who recover may be left with residual brain damage. There may be some degree of paralysis or muscular weakness, difficulties with speech or mental confusion. Hence, recovery and rehabilitation are likely to take some time.

Causes and risk factors: the commonest cause of subarachnoid haemorrhage is accidental head injury. Other causes are rupture of an aneurysm, with atherosclerosis and high blood pressure being significant contributory factors. After a subarachnoid haemorrhage there is a risk of raised intracranial pressure and hydrocephalus.

subdural haemorrhage and haematoma (acute and chronic)

Description: bleeding or haemorrhage that occurs into the space between the outer (dura mater) and middle (arachnoid mater) membranes that surround the brain, causing a collection or clot of blood, a haematoma. An acute subdural haematoma is a common occurrence following a serious head in-

jury and occurs soon after the event. A chronic subdural haematoma may occur some weeks after a
seemingly trivial head injury. The following relates
to the chronic condition.

Persons most commonly affected: adults of both
sexes aged over 50 years but can occur at any age.

Organ or part of body involved: brain.

Symptoms and indications: symptoms may not arise
until some weeks after a relatively minor head injury. They include worsening headaches that occur
each day, periods of drowsiness and confusion,
muscular weakness on one side of the body. In babies, there may be an enlargement of the head if
the haematoma is large. A person with symptoms
of a subdural haematoma requires immediate emergency medical treatment.

Treatment: involves admittance to hospital where
diagnostic tests and scans will first be carried out.
Surgery is then needed to remove the clot and relieve the compression of the brain that is responsible for the symptoms. Once pressure is relieved,
the brain may slowly recover or there may be some
permanent damage. The outlook is best in those
patients who receive prompt surgical intervention.

Causes and risk factors: the cause is previous
trauma to the head that results in internal bleeding,
even though the injury may appear to have been

minor. The risk is greatest in older people or in those who abuse alcohol. There is a risk of death or permanent disability but other patients make a good recovery.

suffocation *see* ASPHYXIA

thromboembolism

Description: the situation in which a blood clot (thrombus) forms in one part of the circulation, usually a vein in the leg (phlebothrombosis), and a portion breaks off and becomes lodged elsewhere, causing a total blockage (embolism). The embolism often involves the pulmonary artery (to the lung) or one of its branches, and this is known as a pulmonary embolism.

Persons most commonly affected: adults of all age groups and both sexes.

Organ or part of body involved: arteries anywhere in the body.

Symptoms and indications: the symptoms depend upon the site of the embolism. In a limb or extremity, symptoms include numbness and tingling, pain and weakness and a weak pulse. In the brain there are symptoms of stroke that vary in severity. In the kidneys, there are symptoms of kidney failure and high blood pressure. If the gastrointestinal tract is involved, there is severe pain, nausea and vomiting, and shock may occur. (*See also* pulmonary embolism.) A person with the symptoms of thromboembolism requires emergency medical treatment. *Treatment*: involves admittance to hospital and, possibly, surgery to remove the clot or bypass a damaged artery. Drugs that may be prescribed include anticoagulants, aspirin and vasodilators to widen blood vessels. Many patients are prescribed anticoagulant drugs before and after planned surgery to lessen the risk of thromboembolism. The condition may prove fatal, depending upon the part of the body that is affected but in other cases it can be cured.

Causes and risk factors: the cause is a blood clot or part of a blood clot that forms in a vein and travels in the circulation to lodge in an artery. The risk increases with conditions such as hypertension (high blood pressure), atherosclerosis, increased age, diabetes mellitus, surgery, injury to blood vessels, pregnancy, smoking, disorders of the circulatory system and a previous history of thromboembolism.

thrombosis (deep vein)

Description: the process of clotting within a vein so that the vessel becomes partially or completely blocked by the clot or thrombus. There is a risk of the clot breaking away and travelling to the lung to cause a pulmonary embolism.

Persons most commonly affected: adults of both sexes.

Organ or part of body involved: veins, especially the deep veins of the calves (lower legs).

Symptoms and indications: symptoms include pain, swelling, tenderness, warmth, redness and the superficial veins may become enlarged and prominent. However, this condition can occur with few or no symptoms, as the lower legs are served by three main veins and thrombosis in one does not affect the functioning of the others. The person usually experiences pain on walking or standing still, which disappears when resting with the leg raised. A person with symptoms of deep vein thrombosis requires immediate medical treatment.

Treatment: the person usually needs to be admitted to hospital for tests, including venography (or phlebography), which produces X-ray images of veins using injected radio-opaque dye. Treatment is by means of anticoagulant drugs, usually heparin, given intravenously, followed by coumarin taken by mouth. The condition can usually be successfully treated, provided that pulmonary embolism does not occur. A person who has had this condition may be advised to wear elasticated stockings, to rest with the feet and lower legs raised, and to avoid sitting with the feet or legs crossed.

Causes and risk factors: the cause of deep vein thrombosis is probably a combination of factors, including damage to the lining of the vein, a pooling of blood due to a decrease in the rate of flow and an increase in the clotting tendency. Risks increase with prolonged bed rest, as occurs after serious illness, injuries or surgery, immediately following childbirth, smoking, taking oral contraceptives and long journeys (especially by air), when a person is sitting for an extended period of time. A person who has to be confined to bed should try to move the legs as much as possible. People who are to undergo planned surgery are frequently given small doses of anticoagulants to lessen the risk of thrombosis.

torsion of a testis or testicle

Description: twisting or rotation of the spermatic cord and testicle, leading to irreversible damage if not treated promptly.

Persons most commonly affected: young adolescent males between the ages of 12 and 20 but can occur at any age.

Organ or part of body involved: testicle – usually only one is affected.

Symptoms and indications: the symptoms may arise for no apparent cause or as a result of strenuous physical activity. Symptoms include severe pain in the testicle, hardening, swelling and reddening of the scrotum, nausea and vomiting, fever and sweating, raised heartbeat rate. A person with these symptoms requires emergency treatment in hospital.

Treatment: is by means of surgery to correct the torsion and to attach the testicle to the wall of the scrotum to prevent a recurrence. Often, the unaffected testicle is similarly fixed at the same time as a precaution. Provided that prompt surgical treatment is carried out, recovery is normally good.

Causes and risk factors: the cause is not known but is sometimes present at birth. If treatment is delayed, the blood supply to the testicle is interrupted, leading to irreversible damage. If this occurs, the testicle and spermatic cord are removed by surgery. The remaining testicle produces sufficient hormones to ensure sexual maturation and fertility.

toxic shock syndrome

Description: a state of acute shock, due to a form of BLOOD POISONING, caused by toxins (poisons) produced by staphylococcal bacteria. The syndrome is generally associated with the use of tampons by women during menstruation, but it may arise for other reasons in males as well as females. It is a rare occurrence, whatever the cause.

Persons most commonly affected: females during menstruation but can affect people of both sexes and all age groups.

Organ or part of body involved: respiratory system, blood, organs.

Symptoms and indications: symptoms include a sudden high fever, diarrhoea, red skin rash, anxiety, headache, fall in blood pressure, mental changes, and confusion and thirst. A person with symptoms of toxic shock syndrome requires emergency medical treatment.

Treatment: involves admittance to hospital for intensive supportive nursing. The person requires high doses of antibiotics (especially penicillin and cephalosporin), fluids and electrolytes all given intravenously until symptoms subside. The condition can be cured if caught and treated early but may prove fatal in some cases.

Causes and risk factors: the cause is toxins released by staphylococcus bacteria into the blood circulation. The syndrome can arise as a result of an infection within the body or from a wound, as well as from the use of tampons. Women should wash their hands before and after the insertion of a tampon and change tampons frequently. It is thought that young women or girls in whom the immune system is not fully developed may be at greater risk, particularly if a tampon is left in place too long.

transient ischaemic attack (TIA)

Description: a temporary decrease in the normal supply of blood to a part of the brain. Usually the artery involved is partially blocked by a small plaque of material due to atherosclerosis, or a blood clot or embolus.

Persons most commonly affected: middle-aged and elderly adults of both sexes but can affect younger people and children with heart and circulatory disease.

Organ or part of body involved: one of the arteries supplying the brain, especially a branch of the carotid artery (in the neck) or the vertebral-basilar system of arteries.

Symptoms and indications: symptoms come on abruptly and last for two minutes to one or two hours (rarely longer). They include muscular weakness and numbness or tingling in the limbs, disturbance of vision or loss of sight in one eye, slurred speech or loss of the ability to speak, giddiness and confusion. The person remains conscious throughout the episode. Attacks tend to recur and vary in frequency from two or three each day to one or two over several years. A person with symptoms of a transient ischaemic attack should seek medical advice.

Treatment: depends, to a certain extent, upon the patient's condition and whether any underlying disorders are discovered or known to be present. The person is likely to be examined for high blood pressure (hypertension), diabetes mellitus, and heart disease, and a blood sample may be taken to check for raised levels of fats (lipids) and polycythaemia (an abnormal increase in the number of red blood cells). If the attack is an isolated one or a rare occurrence, the person is usually treated with a small daily dose of aspirin. For more frequent attacks, anticoagulants such as heparin may be prescribed, or antiplatelet drugs. Some patients may require surgery to remove atherosclerotic deposits or plaques from a carotid artery. A person who experiences a transient ischaemic attack should have regular medical check-ups and monitoring.

Causes and risk factors: the cause of the condition is a partial temporary blockage of an artery supplying the brain by a fatty deposit, piece of arterial wall or blood clot. The risk increases in those who smoke, who are obese or who have high blood pressure, diabetes mellitus, high levels of cholesterol or other fats in the blood, atherosclerosis or polycythaemia. There is an increased risk of stroke in those who have transient ischaemic attacks and treatment is aimed at preventing the occurrence of this serious condition. A stroke is probably more likely to occur in a person who does not receive treatment for a transient ischaemic attack.